SpringerBriefs in Applied Sciences and Technology

SpringerBriefs present concise summaries of cutting-edge research and practical applications across a wide spectrum of fields. Featuring compact volumes of 50 to 125 pages, the series covers a range of content from professional to academic.

Typical publications can be:

- A timely report of state-of-the art methods
- An introduction to or a manual for the application of mathematical or computer techniques
- A bridge between new research results, as published in journal articles
- A snapshot of a hot or emerging topic
- An in-depth case study
- A presentation of core concepts that students must understand in order to make independent contributions

SpringerBriefs are characterized by fast, global electronic dissemination, standard publishing contracts, standardized manuscript preparation and formatting guidelines, and expedited production schedules.

On the one hand, **SpringerBriefs in Applied Sciences and Technology** are devoted to the publication of fundamentals and applications within the different classical engineering disciplines as well as in interdisciplinary fields that recently emerged between these areas. On the other hand, as the boundary separating fundamental research and applied technology is more and more dissolving, this series is particularly open to trans-disciplinary topics between fundamental science and engineering.

Indexed by EI-Compendex, SCOPUS and Springerlink.

Tin-Chih Toly Chen

Explainable Ambient Intelligence (XAmI)

Explainable Artificial Intelligence Applications in Smart Life

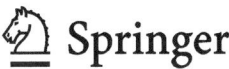 Springer

Tin-Chih Toly Chen 🆔
Industrial Engineering and Management
National Yang Ming Chiao Tung University
Hsinchu, Taiwan

ISSN 2191-530X   ISSN 2191-5318 (electronic)
SpringerBriefs in Applied Sciences and Technology
ISBN 978-3-031-54934-2   ISBN 978-3-031-54935-9 (eBook)
https://doi.org/10.1007/978-3-031-54935-9

This Springer imprint is published by the registered company Springer Nature Switzerland AG
The registered company address is: Gewerbestrasse 11, 6330 Cham, Switzerland

Paper in this product is recyclable.

Contents

1 **Ambient Intelligence (AmI)** 1
  1.1 Ambient Intelligence (AmI) 1
  1.2 Architecture and Operational Procedure of AmI Systems 3
  1.3 Examples of AmI Applications 4
  1.4 Issues and Challenges of Existing AmI Applications 7
  1.5 Artificial Intelligence (AI) for Enhancing the Effectiveness
     of AmI Applications 8
  1.6 Explainable Ambient Intelligence (XAmI): Explainable
     Artificial Intelligence (XAI) Applications to AmI 9
  1.7 Examples of XAmI Applications 10
  1.8 Organization of This Book 15
  References 17

2 **Explainable Artificial Intelligence (XAI) with Applications** 23
  2.1 Explainable Artificial Intelligence (XAI) 23
  2.2 Explainability of ML Models 24
  2.3 XAI for Explaining and Enhancing AI Applications
     in Ambient Intelligence (AmI) 24
  2.4 Requirements for Trustable AI and XAI 26
  2.5 Classification of XAI Methods 27
  2.6 XAI Applications in Various Domains 29
  2.7 Types of Explanations 30
  2.8 XAI Techniques for Feature Importance Evaluation 33
  References 35

3 **XAmI Applications to Smart Homes** 39
  3.1 Artificial Intelligence (AI) Applications in Smart Homes 39
  3.2 XAmI Technique for Explaining Fuzzy Logic Applications
     in Smart Homes 48

3.3   XAmI Technique for Explaining ANN Applications in Smart
      Homes 49
      3.3.1   Interpretable Model-Agnostic Explanation (LIME) 49
      3.3.2   LIME + Decision Trees (DTs) 50
      3.3.3   LIME + Random Forests (RFs) 52
      3.3.4   LIME + Fuzzy Inference Rules 53
      References 58

4   **XAmI Applications to Location-Aware Services** 63
    4.1   Artificial Intelligence (AI) Applications in Location-Aware
          Services (LASs) 63
    4.2   Issues of Existing AI Applications in LASs 65
    4.3   XAmI Applications in Location-Aware Services 65
          4.3.1   Suitable XAmI Methods for Location-Aware Services 65
          4.3.2   Various Types of Explanations for Location-Aware
                  Services 68
          4.3.3   Visualization XAmI Methods for Location-Aware
                  Services 70
    4.4   Criteria Priority Versus Impact 77
    4.5   Explaining AI-Based Optimization in LASs 78
          4.5.1   Local and Contrastive Explanations for AI-Based
                  Optimization in LASs 78
    References 80

5   **XAmI Applications to Telemedicine and Telecare** 85
    5.1   Artificial Intelligence (AI) Applications in Telemedicine
          and Telecare 85
    5.2   Effectiveness of AI Applications for Telemedicine
          and Telecare Services 88
    5.3   Explainable Ambient Intelligence (XAmI) Applications
          in Telemedicine and Telecare 91
    5.4   Popular XAmI Techniques for Telemedicine and Telecare 93
          5.4.1   SHAP 93
          5.4.2   LIME with Decision Tree (DT) Application 96
          5.4.3   LIME with Random Forest (RF) Application 99
    5.5   Applicability Assessment of Telemedicine and Telecare
          Services Based on XAmI 101
    5.6   Issues with Existing XAmI Applications in Telemedicine
          and Telecare 103
    References 105

Chapter 1
Ambient Intelligence (AmI)

Abstract This chapter begins by defining ambient intelligence (AmI). The chronology of the emergence of the most widely used AmI technologies is then provided. Through reviewing some cases in the literature, AmI applications prevalent in various fields are mentioned, such as emotionally pleasing design, telemedicine and telecare, context-aware recommendation, home care and assisted living, smart home, smart tourism, and smart factory. The issues and challenges that need to be addressed by existing AmI applications are then discussed. To solve these problems and challenges, the most popular artificial intelligence (AI) technologies are highlighted. However, some AI technologies are very complex, limiting the interpretability and credibility of related AmI applications. To address this problem, the combination of AmI and XAI results in XAmI, and a review of some existing XAmI applications is performed. Based on the review findings, the application of XAmI techniques and tools is expected to mitigate the social impacts of AI applications in AmI on fairness and bias, security, verifiability, and accountability.

Keywords Ambient intelligence · Artificial intelligence · Explainable artificial intelligence · Explainable ambient intelligence

1.1 Ambient Intelligence (AmI)

Ambient Intelligence (AmI) is the vision of an environment supporting users in an unobtrusive/transparent, interconnected, adaptive, dynamic, embedded, and intelligent way [1–2]. In this vision, environments are sensitive to the needs of their inhabitants and able to anticipate their needs and behaviors [3–4]. AmI systems come in many forms, such as smart homes, smart factories, smart stores, mobility guides, virtual tours, ubiquitous healthcare systems, online social networks, telemedicine, and telecare. The key to the success of an AmI system is the perception and interpretation of user needs [5]. To achieve this, human factors and ergonomics (HFE) is a useful tool [6].

© The Author(s), under exclusive license to Springer Nature Switzerland AG 2024
T.-C. T. Chen, *Explainable Ambient Intelligence (XAmI)*,
SpringerBriefs in Applied Sciences and Technology,
https://doi.org/10.1007/978-3-031-54935-9_1

The concept of AmI was proposed in 2001. Over the years, many AmI applications have become more common and less expensive (see Fig. 1.1). Today, smart switches that can be controlled via a remote smartphone cost less than $100. However, after years of attempts, some AmI applications have proven unsuccessful, such as smart clothing, which is one of the key technologies for telemedicine [7–8]. Until recently, technological, cultural, and market conditions did not support the widespread adoption of smart clothing [9–10]. In contrast, taking smart homes as an example, the global smart home market was estimated to be US$80.21 billion in 2022 and is expected to grow from US$93.98 billion in 2023 to US$338.28 billion in 2030 [11].

The COVID-19 pandemic has brought about dramatic changes in the applications of AmI technologies. AmI technologies applied during the COVID-19 pandemic differed from those applied before the outbreak (see Fig. 1.2). According to Chen and Wang's observations [12], users' motivations for applying AmI technologies have also changed. Before the outbreak of COVID-19, AmI technology applications were called for better **smart life**. In contrast, applications during the pandemic were mainly about avoiding infection (i.e., preventing disease), that is, focusing on **distant healthcare**.

In **location-aware services (LASs)**, applications were designed to help find where to buy masks, remind users to wear masks, or detect whether users were wearing masks. In **telecare**, most applications developed during this period were used to provide information or news about COVID-19, record symptoms, and contact tracing. In **smart home**, smart watches were used to track people's health (including heart rate and sleep time) and physical activity (including gestures, movements, steps, and movements), since people stayed at home longer. In **smart tourism**, hotel visitors felt more at ease if robots provided services during the pandemic. Additionally,

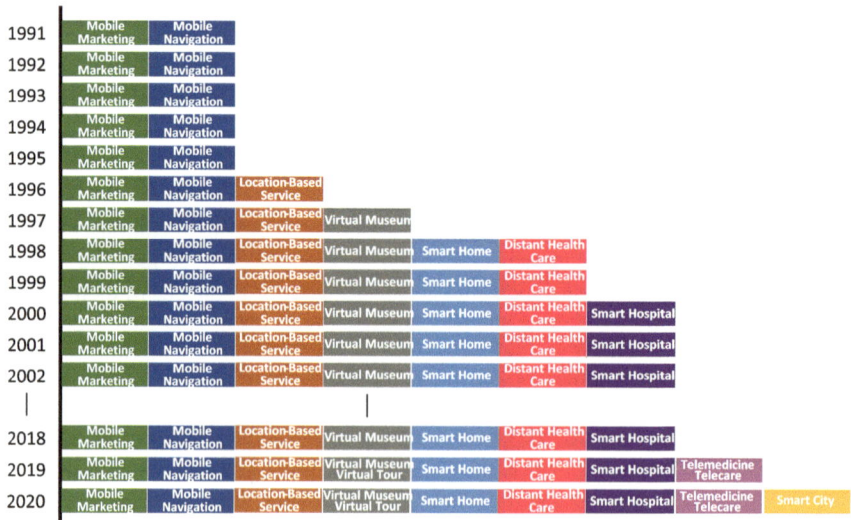

Fig. 1.1 Emergence of AmI applications

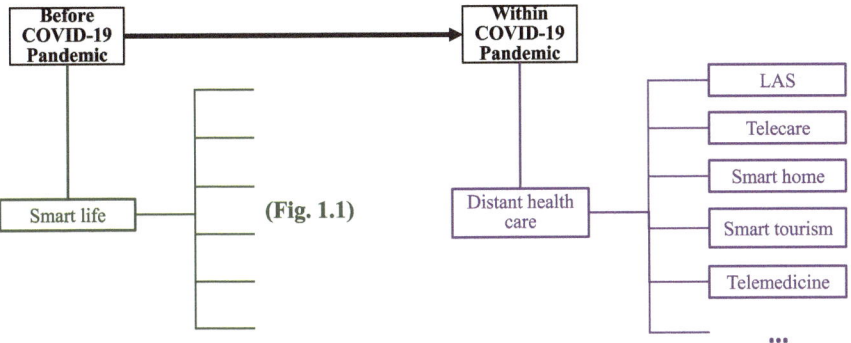

Fig. 1.2 Comparison of AmI technologies applied before and during the COVID-19 pandemic

in **telemedicine**, the GPS tracker on a smart bracelet or sociometric badge helped measure a patient's temperature and blood oxygen levels, ensuring the patient's commitment to isolation and social distancing.

1.2   Architecture and Operational Procedure of AmI Systems

Cook et al. [13] established an AmI system architecture containing four layers. Figure 1.3 shows how various disciplines map to the four layers [14].

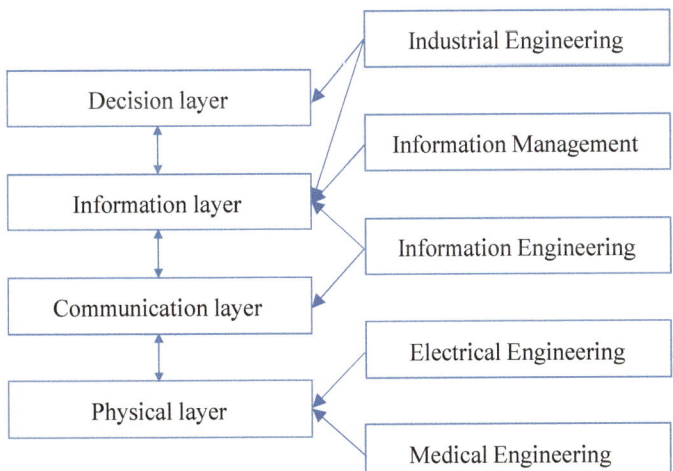

Fig. 1.3 Mapping various disciplines to the four layers of an AmI system

Fig. 1.4 Systematic
procedure for constructing
AmI systems or providing
related services

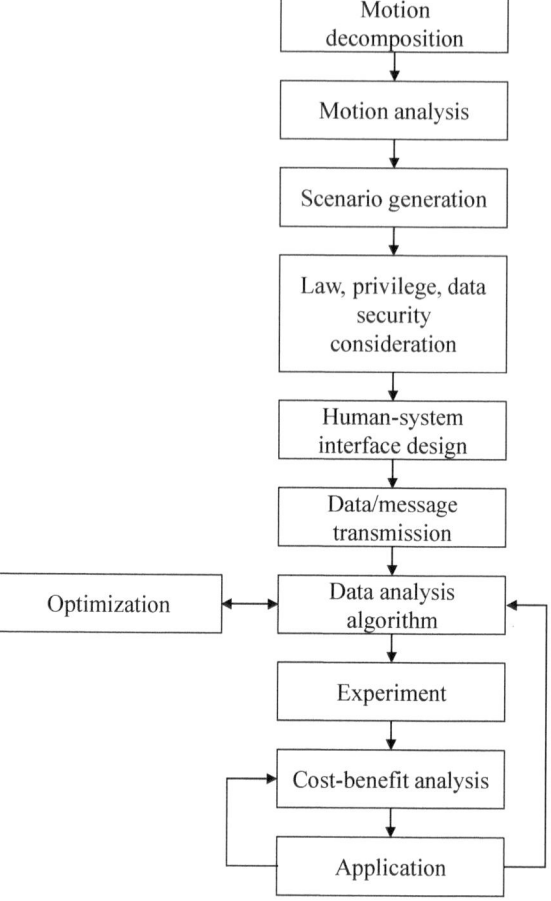

Chen [15] established a systematic procedure for constructing AmI systems or providing related services (see Fig. 1.4).

1.3 Examples of AmI Applications

In **affective and pleasurable design**, easy-to-understand algorithms need to be identified so that designers can use to create novel concept designs. Wang and Yang [16] selected popular motorcycles as sample products and used the most distinctive front handle covers as design targets. Their affective and pleasurable design approach consisted of three stages: preparation, construction of conceptual creativity, and semantic analysis. After comparing random sketches of ideas with existing designs on the market, they found that some of the conceptual designs obtained using the proposed approach were very innovative and could easily be redesigned for actual products.

Otebolaku and Andrade [17] studied **context-aware recommendation** techniques for implicitly delivering context-sensitive online media items. The proposed recommendation service identified a user's dynamic contextual situation from built-in sensors and used case-based reasoning (CBR) [18] to determine the user's current contextual preferences. The effectiveness of the proposed recommendation service was evaluated through a case study.

For a similar purpose, Van den Auld et al. [19] built a convolutional neural network (CNN) to recommend suitable music to users. The inputs and output of the DNN were the favorite clips of a piece of music and the category of the music, respectively. Then the trained CNN was used to classify a new piece of music. For users who have not heard similar music, recommendations were made based on latent factors.

Wang et al. [20] built a deep neural network (DNN) to help diagnose users with type-II diabetes through an application in a **telemedicine** service. The physical conditions entered by the user were transmitted to the backend server where the DNN resided. However, although the diagnostic results were easy to understand, the diagnostic mechanism was difficult for users to figure out.

A research trend in AmI is to identify the types of **quality of life** that are more relevant to users and to develop actions to improve these qualities of life. For example, Chen [21] argued that acceptability, efficiency, and immediacy are three key types of quality of life for patients who are mobile and looking for a suitable clinic. In order to optimize these types of quality of life as a whole, ordered weighted average (OWA) [22–23] is applied to aggregate the performances of a clinic in multiple dimensions. In addition, increasing the comfort of mobile users by joining online social networks has attracted increasing attention from researchers [24].

Smart life and smart world are extensions of smart home and are also important applications of AmI. Pisula and Kossakowska [25] fit the relationship between the sense of coherence (including understandability, manageability, and meaningfulness) and the quality of life of parents of autistic children in smart families. In contrast, previous studies have primarily considered fear, stress, independence, communication, and social support [26–28]. Gao et al. [29] considered temporal information to improve the quality of life of mobile users by joining online social networks, while previous studies only considered spatial and social information [30–32].

Domestic care and **assisted living** for the elderly are important applications for AmI. Thakur and Han [33] built a human behavior monitoring system in which user interactions were semantically analyzed by considering different situational parameters during daily life activities to identify a list of different behavior patterns related to various activities. Furthermore, a novel decision-making algorithm was also proposed to analyze these behavioral patterns and their relationship with the dynamic situational and spatial characteristics of the environment to detect any anomalies in user behavior that may constitute an emergency situation.

Smart tourism is a special application field of AmI [34]. In this field, information technology (IT) empowers the creation of novel travel experiences and increasingly adds value to all stages of travel. Smart environments (such as smart museums, smart libraries, smart theaters, and smart department stores) have changed the structure of the tourism industry, as well as people's travel methods and processes [35]. The service strategy, management, marketing, and competitiveness of each relevant participant have also been disrupted.

After the end of 2020, as COVID-19 vaccinations became widespread and people began to resume regional tourism, outdoor attractions such as recreational agricultural parks were particularly attractive because they were well-ventilated and could prevent the spread of COVID-19. However, during the COVID-19 pandemic, considerations surrounding choosing a recreational agricultural park were different than usual and subject to uncertainty. Therefore, Wu et al. [36] proposed a fuzzy collaborative intelligence (FCI) approach to help select recreational agricultural parks suitable for traveler groups during the COVID-19 pandemic. The proposed FCI approach combined asymmetric calibrated fuzzy geometric mean (acFGM), fuzzy weighted intersection (FWI), and fuzzy Vise Kriterijumska Optimizacija I Kompromisno Resenje (fuzzy VIKOR). The experimental results showed that travelers (especially traveler groups) were very willing to go to leisure agricultural parks during the COVID-19 pandemic. In addition, the most important criterion for selecting a suitable leisure agricultural park was whether it was easy to maintain social distance, while the least important criterion was the distance to the leisure agricultural park.

In Costa et al. [37], the emotions of family members were detected through smart wristbands to determine the required environmental changes. After being transmitted to the smart home console, **smart home** appliances can change the home environment to try to achieve specific emotions. (e.g., calm or excited). Caregivers can also be notified if necessary. Fall detection is another key feature of smart homes and assisted living. Due to the rapid development of sensor networks and the Internet of things (IoT), human–machine interaction using sensor fusion has been considered an effective method to solve the fall detection problem. By detecting and classifying resident movements, possible falls can be predicted and/or prevented, which requires the use of XAI technologies to explain the prediction process and results.

Advances in **telemedicine and telecare** technologies improve the ubiquitous healthcare environment. One of the key applications is a ubiquitous clinic recommendation system, which recommends suitable clinics to a mobile patient based on his/her location, required specialty, and preferences. However, patients may be unwilling or unable to express their preferences. To overcome this problem, some ubiquitous clinic recommender systems mine patients' historical data to learn their preferences and adjust their recommendation algorithms as they receive more patient data. This adjustment mechanism may operate for several periods, but may not last forever. In order to solve this problem, Chiu and Chiu [38] modeled the improvement of the successful recommendation rate of a ubiquitous clinic recommendation system. The adjustment mechanism of the ubiquitous clinic recommendation system is considered to be a learning process [39–41], in which both the asymptotic value and learning speed of the learning process provide valuable information that can help improve the long-term effectiveness of the adjustment mechanism [42]. The proposed methodology adapted the ubiquitous clinic recommendation mechanism by rollingly solving an integer-nonlinear programming (INLP) problem.

The COVID-19 pandemic has severely affected factories around the world, which have closed to avoid the spread of COVID-19. Ensuring long-term factory operations during the COVID-19 pandemic therefore becomes a critical but challenging task. To accomplish this task, the application of smart and automated technologies is considered an effective means. However, such applications are time-consuming and budget-intensive, have varying effectiveness, and may not necessarily be acceptable to workers. In order to make full use of limited resources and time, it is necessary to establish a systematic procedure to compare various applications of smart and automation technologies. To this end, Chen and Lin [43] proposed an evolving fuzzy assessment approach. First, the alpha-cut operations (ACO) [44]-fuzzy analytic hierarchy process (FAHP) [10] method was used, based on the judgment of factory managers, to derive the priorities of criteria for evaluating the applications of smart and automation technologies to ensure long-term operations during the COVID-19 pandemic. In this step, in order to improve the calculation efficiency of ACO, a genetic algorithm (GA) was designed. Subsequently, fuzzy technique for order preference by similarity to an ideal solution (FTOPSIS) was applied to evaluate the overall effectiveness of each smart and automation technology application based on the derived priorities. Smart and automation technology applications with the best performance were selected. They studied the case of a **smart factory** to demonstrate the effectiveness of the evolving fuzzy assessment approach in ensuring the long-term operation during the COVID-19 pandemic.

Three-dimensional (3D) printing has great potential for establishing a ubiquitous service in telemedicine. However, the planning, optimization, and control of a ubiquitous 3D printing network have not been sufficiently discussed. Therefore, Wang et al. [45] established a collaborative and ubiquitous system for making dental parts using 3D printing. After an order of dental parts was received, the collaborative and ubiquitous system split the order among nearby 3D printing facilities to fulfill the order collaboratively and formed a delivery plan to pick up the 3D-printed dental parts. To optimize the performances of the two tasks, a mixed integer linear programming (MILP) model and a mixed integer quadratic programming (MIQP) model were optimized respectively. In addition, slack information was derived and provided to each 3D printing facility so that it can determine the feasibility of resuming the same 3D printing process locally from the beginning without violating the optimality of the original printing and delivery plan. Further, more slack was gained by considering the chain effect between two successive 3D printing facilities.

1.4 Issues and Challenges of Existing AmI Applications

There are several issues and challenges that need to be addressed for AmI applications. First, some AmI systems have not yet been implemented on a commercial basis [46–47], and many of them have never undergone a cost–benefit analysis [48–49]. One of the reasons for this is large-scale government supports, which is not focused on profits, but another reason is the difficulty in collecting cost and benefit information on the customer and user side [50–51]. For example, a user may use the restaurant recommendation system but not go to the recommended restaurant [52–53], resulting in costs on the system side, which represents a system failure, although the user has made a decision based on the information provided by the restaurant recommendation system. Benefits like this can be difficult to measure because the system does not receive commissions from recommended restaurants [54–55]. In addition, it is difficult to connect the user's final decision with the recommendation given. To make AmI systems sustainable, a reliable cost–benefit analysis is necessary, which requires overcoming these issues [56–57].

Secondly, although AmI applications can be modeled as a human–machine interaction process, in which human factors and ergonomics are an integral part and should be taken seriously, most AmI-related research is conducted by researchers with information engineering, electrical engineering, and information engineering, management, and medicine backgrounds, rather than ergonomics [58–60].

AmI systems can overcome these problems and pursue sustainable development through the following methods: constantly updating the database, adding new features and eliminating old or unpopular services, providing users with more choices and flexibility, researching ways to increase profits, and improving applicability to users [48, 61–62].

1.5 Artificial Intelligence (AI) for Enhancing the Effectiveness of AmI Applications

To enhance the effectiveness of AmI applications, artificial intelligence (AI) technologies have been widely applied in this field. AmI can also be considered as an emerging branch of AI with user-centric applications. AmI is also an interdisciplinary challenge for researchers with backgrounds in information engineering, electrical engineering, and medicine [63]. AmI applications also face the same difficulties encountered by other AI applications. More and more deep learning (DL) techniques are being applied to AmI, but these DL techniques are far from being well understood [64]. Less explainable AI methods, the so-called black boxes, include artificial neural networks (ANNs) [65–66], fuzzy neural systems [67], DL, random forest (RF) [68–69], advanced fuzzy logic [70–71], support vector machines [72–73], bio-inspired algorithms (such as GAs [74–75] and artificial bee colony (ABC) [76]), agent-based systems [77–78], and others [79].

Figure 1.5 provides statistics on the popularity of AI technology applications in AmI. AI technologies most widely used in AmI include deep learning, fuzzy neural systems, and agent-based systems.

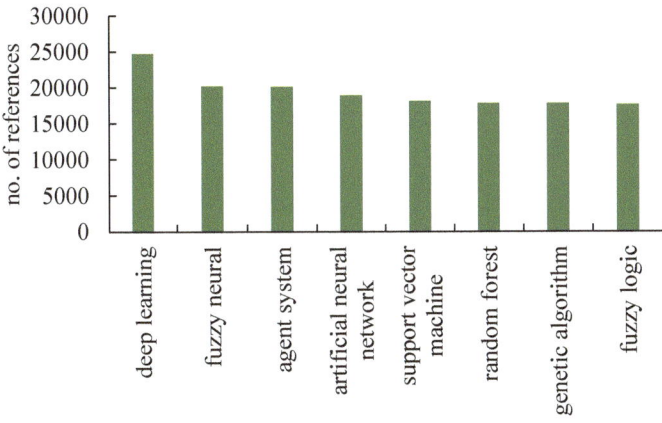

Fig. 1.5 Number of references about AI technology applications in AmI from 2010 to 2023 (Data source Google Scholar)

1.6 Explainable Ambient Intelligence (XAmI): Explainable Artificial Intelligence (XAI) Applications to AmI

AI applications have penetrated into every aspect of AmI. However, the applied AI technologies are becoming increasingly complex, limiting the interpretability and credibility of related AmI applications [80]. Explainable artificial intelligence (XAI) is to enhance the practicality of an existing AI technology by explaining its reasoning process and/or result [81–84].

Cassens and Wegener [85] argued that AmI is specifically poised to support technology developments that drive ethics and transparency due to the paradigmatic imperatives of system intelligence, social intelligence, and embeddedness. They also argued that the AmI systems are well suited for inferring when an explanation is needed (and what type of explanation) and what form it should take. They further proposed that AmI devices serve as intermediaries between humans and machines, combining social and technical systems in a fully embedded manner.

The societal impacts of AI include: fairness and bias, safety, verifiability, and accountability, as summarized in Table 1.1 [86–88]. As the table shows, the application of XAI techniques and tools is expected to mitigate these impacts, especially in the domain of AmI, as described below.

LASs are a common application of AmI [32, 53]. A restaurant recommendation app can be unethical because it directs users to restaurants that are advertised on the app, rather than strictly following the user's request. Most LAS systems will require users to feedback on their choices, so as to verify the effectiveness of the recommendation mechanism in terms of the successful recommendation rate [78, 89]. In addition, an automatic driving system, as an advanced human–machine interface, is also an important function of AmI [90]. However, due to immature software and hardware technologies, automatic driving systems are still unsafe and may cause

Table 1.1 Societal impacts of AI

Societal impact of AI	Description	XAI application
Fairness and bias	The algorithm used in an AI system may be unfair or unethical	• Bias detection • Bias mitigation • Bias explainability • Simulation to understand long-term impact of algorithm
Safety	AI systems should not inadvertently or maliciously make decisions or take actions that are unsafe to humans	XAI helps identify fail states in the model (that lead to danger)
Verifiability	Verifiability helps identify cases where an AI system mail fail or not have an explanation	With explainability, the verification of an AI system can be formulated as a computationally tractable optimization problem
Accountability	Accountability is the ability to acknowledge and attribute responsibility for decisions made by an AI system	XAI techniques and tools for approximating the relationship between the inputs and output

accidents to users [91]. In a self-health management application, a DNN can be built on the backend server to diagnose whether a user has type-II diabetes according to the attributes entered by the user. However, the diagnostic mechanism is far beyond the user's understanding. Therefore, the diagnostic mechanism of the DNN is usually approximated with simpler decision rules to explain the results to users [19].

Therefore, Kamath and Liu [86] argued that XAI applications can improve our society and build a better world. It is foreseeable that the applications of XAI in the field of AmI will spawn a large number of **explainable ambient intelligence (XAmI)** applications.

1.7 Examples of XAmI Applications

In the field of telemedicine, Wang et al. [19] built an ANN to diagnose patients with type-II diabetes, where a patient could access the ANN running on the server (or doctor) side using an app on his/her smartphone. Some of the inputs to the ANN had to be entered by the patient on the client side, while other inputs were retrieved from the patient's medical record in the hospital information system. To facilitate communication of diagnostic processes and results with patients, **decision trees** (DTs) [22] (see Fig. 1.6) are used to approximate the ANN, following the concept of **Locally Interpretable Model-Agnostic Explanations (LIME)** [92–93]. Another XAI tool for building and visualizing the ANN is TensorFlow (see Fig. 1.7).

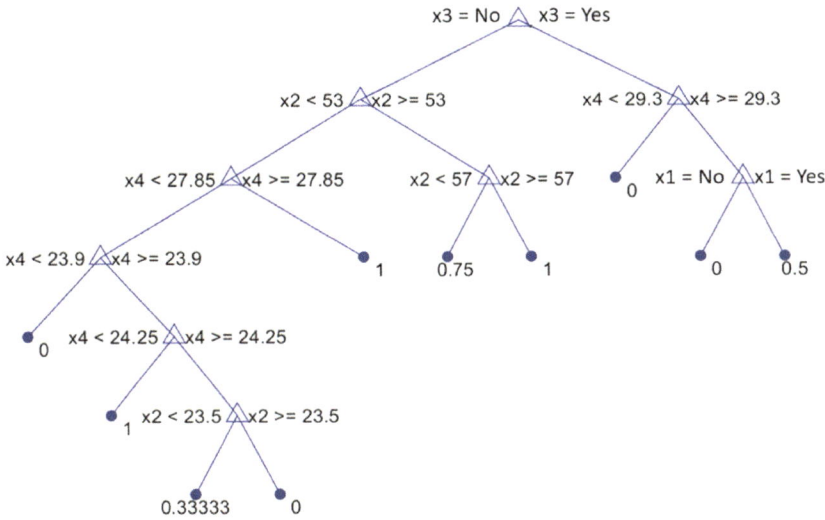

Fig. 1.6 DT for explaining an ANN application in type-II diabetes diagnosis

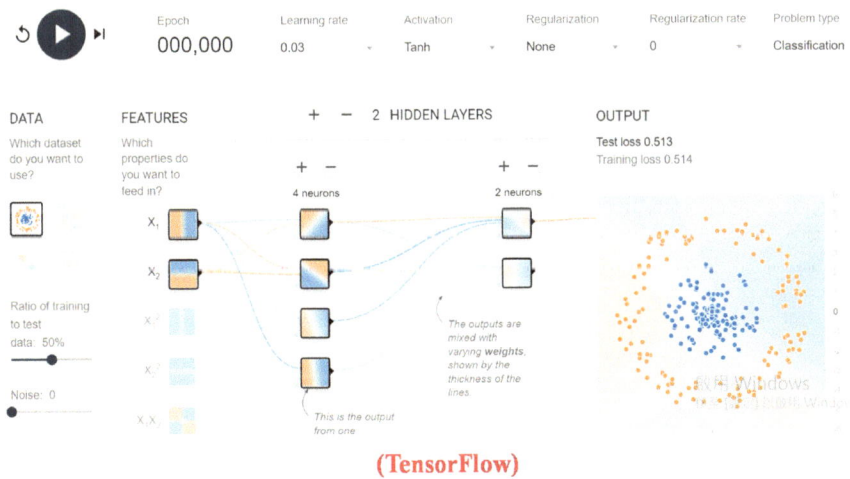

Fig. 1.7 TensorFlow for building and visualizing the ANN application

Moulouel et al. [94] proposed a hybrid method combining deep learning and probabilistic common-sense reasoning to predict human activities in AmI environments, where deep learning models were built to identify environmental objects, human hands, and the user's indoor location. The probabilistic flow was then introduced into the formalism of event calculus formulated in **answer set programming (ECASP)**. Inference axioms were based on ontologies that described the context in which users perform activities. Through reasoning based on time projection and abduction, the proposed methodology enabled the XAI interpretation of activity expectations.

During the COVID-19 pandemic, it was difficult for travelers to choose a suitable nature leisure travel destination because many factors were related to health risks and were highly uncertain. Lin and Chen [95] proposed a type-II fuzzy approach using XAI to overcome this difficulty. First, an innovative type-II alpha-cut operations-fuzzy collaborative intelligence method was used to derive the fuzzy priorities of key factors for nature-based leisure travel destination selection. Subsequently, the type-II fuzzy Vise Kriterijumska Optimizacija I Kompromisno Resenje method was adopted to evaluate and compare the overall performances of nature-based leisure tourism destinations. Additionally, several measures have been taken to enhance the interpretability of the selection process and results, including **color management, common expressions, annotated figures** (Fig. 1.8), **traceable aggregation**, and **segmented distance diagram** [96–97].

Smart factories are another field where AmI technologies are widely used to promote human–machine system interaction. Chen et al. [98] proposed an FCI method to improve the precision of cycle time range estimation, which is an important task in controlling smart factories [99], in which a DNN was first constructed to accurately predict the cycle time of a job, and then a **RF** was built to interpret the DNN. Each decision tree of RF was fuzzified to estimate the cycle time range of the job for which the decision tree was learned. A fuzzy collaboration mechanism was also established between decision trees to reduce the cycle time range.

Fall detection is an important feature for many AmI applications such as smart homes and LASs. Mankodiya et al. [100] jointly used three different sensors for fall detection, which were placed at five different locations on the subject's body to

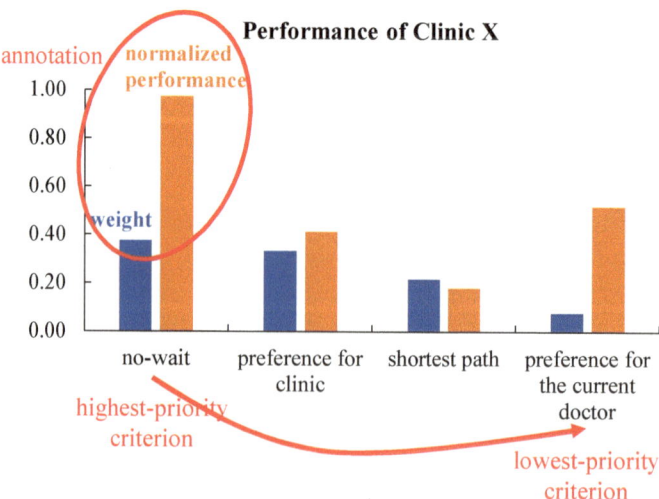

Fig. 1.8 Grouped bar chart illustrating color management, common expressions, and annotated figures

collect the data needed to train AI models for fall detection, which were long short-term memory (LSTM) neural networks and a majority voting classifier was used to determine the final result. In addition to the system architecture and performance (including accuracy, recall, precision, and $F1$) for **global explanations**, **LIME** was also used to provide **local explanations** by evaluating the importance of each input to the output for each user.

Venugopal et al. [101] compared the performances of classifying X-ray images into two states (pneumonia and non-pneumonia) or 14 classes using two AI methods: the pneumonia detection algorithm (using region-based fully convolutional networks, relation networks, and RetinaNets) and Stanford baseline X-ray classification model (using DenseNet121s). To explain and improve the diagnostic performance using the AI applications, **heatmaps** were plotted to show the parts of an X-ray image that was focused on classification.

Many decision-making problems in AmI applications are fuzzy group decision-making tasks. However, when decision-makers lack consensus, existing methods either ignore this fact or force the decision-maker to change his/her judgment. However, these actions may be unreasonable. To solve this problem, Chen and Chiu [52] proposed an XAI-enhanced fuzzy collaborative intelligence method that seeks the consensus among experts in a novel way, in which the fuzzy judgment matrix of each decision-maker was decomposed into multiple fuzzy judgment submatrices. Then, an overall consensus could be easily found from the fuzzy judgment subma-trixed of all decision-makers, for which a **consensus diagram** (see Fig. 1.9) was used to illustrate the process.

XAI techniques and tools have been widely applied in telemedicine or telecare. For example, in the telemedicine system established by Barakat et al. [102] for diagnosing type-II diabetes, support vector machine (SVM) was applied to classify patients as having diabetes or not based on ten demographic or physical characteristics. In addition to plotting and analyzing the receiver operating characteristic (ROC) curve, they also built **DTs** from the classification results. The ROC curves provided a global explanation, while the rules in the DTs were a common intrinsic XAI method that provided a local explanation for each patient. Nagaraj et al. [103] applied four machine learning (ML) methods, namely SVM, RF, decision tree, and extreme gradient boosting (XGBoost), to predict the probability that a user has diabetes. The accuracy was highest when using RF. LIME was then used to explain the prediction process using linear regression (LR) or DTs and make recommendations to the patients accordingly.

The goals of XAmI and tools that are reviewed above for achieving these goals are shown in Fig. 1.10.

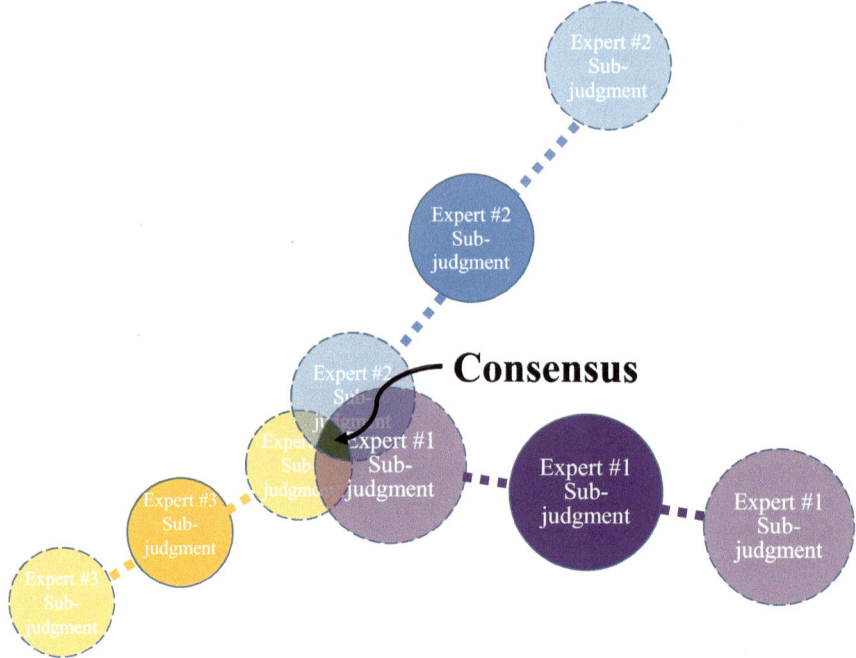

Fig. 1.9 Consensus diagram

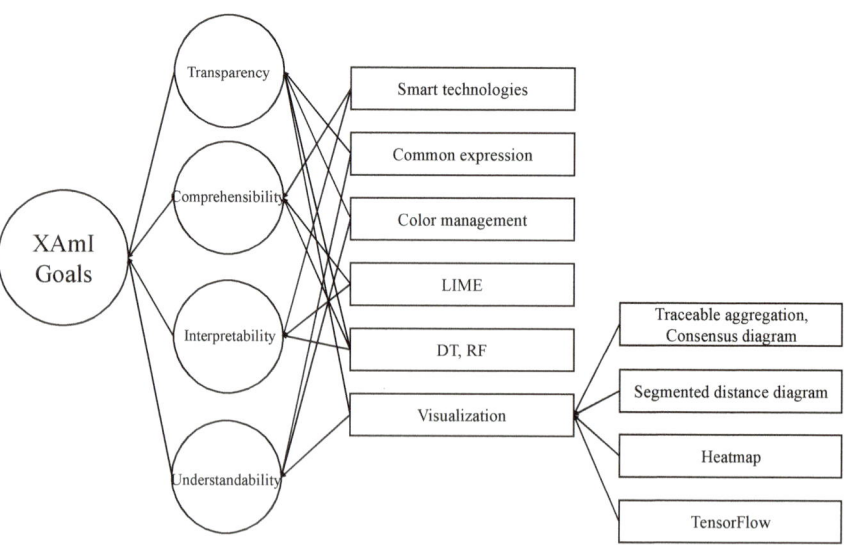

Fig. 1.10 XAmI goals and tools

1.8 Organization of This Book

This book discusses the application of XAI in AmI, the so-called explainable AmI (XAmI): "XAmI is to explain the execution process and/or results of the application of AI technology in AmI." Compared with XAI in other fields, XAmI has the following novel features:

- The applications of XAI technologies and tools in other fields can also be used to explain the applications of AI technologies in the AmI field.
- However, the application subject of XAmI should be users, which is slightly different from the applications of AI technologies in other fields.
- User backgrounds of AmI applications are very diverse. These users may lack relevant knowledge of AI technologies. In contrast, users of AmI applications in manufacturing typically have engineering and management knowledge or skills [104]. Some users of AmI applications, such as healthcare professionals, have medical-related professions.
- XAI is especially needed in high-risk fields such as medical care and credit loans. The risks to users in the AmI field may not be high.
- Understandability and intelligibility mean that system structures and algorithms that require background knowledge are not mentioned when explaining AI applications, so they are more important aspects of XAmI.

This book is dedicated to systematically reviewing the progress of XAmI and introducing XAmI methods, tools, and applications.

In specific, the outline of the present book is structured as follows.

In the current chapter, AmI is first defined. A chronology of the emergence of the most widely used AmI technologies is then detailed. Through some cases in the literature, common AmI technology applications in various fields are mentioned, such as affective and pleasurable design, telemedicine and telecare, context-aware recommendation, LASs, quality of life, smart life, domestic care and assisted living, smart homes, smart tourism, and smart factories. The issues and challenges that AmI applications need to address are then discussed. To solve these problems and challenges, the most popular AI technologies are introduced. However, some AI technologies are very complex, limiting the interpretability and credibility of related AmI applications. To address this problem, the combination of AmI and XAI results in XAmI, and some existing XAmI applications are reviewed. Based on the review findings, the application of XAmI technologies and tools is expected to mitigate the social impacts of AI on fairness and bias, security, verifiability, and accountability.

Chapter 2, Explainable Artificial Intelligence (XAI) with Applications, begins by defining explainable artificial intelligence (XAI). The explainabilities of existing ML models are then compared, showing the need for XAI applications to improve the explainabilities of some ML models. To this end, XAI techniques and tools for interpreting and enhancing artificial intelligence applications, especially in the field of ambient intelligence (AmI), are discussed. Subsequently, the requirements for trustable AI and XAI are listed. Various classifications of existing XAI methods are then performed to meet these requirements. A literature analysis was also conducted on the application of XAI in various fields, showing that services, medicine, and education are the most common application fields of XAI. Finally, several types of explanations are introduced.

Chapter 3, XAmI Applications to Smart Homes, focuses on smart homes where users spend most of their time. However, unlike location-aware systems or telemedicine or telecare systems, smart homes can be controlled by the user, even from the outside. Therefore, assisting users in operating smart home appliances has become a key task. To accomplish this task, various sensors and actuators are installed in smart home appliances to detect user conditions and needs, accompanied by many artificial intelligence (AI) applications. This chapter first summarizes the applications of AI technologies in smart homes. Explainable artificial intelligence (XAI) techniques can then be applied to extract useful behavioral patterns of users from these AI applications, thereby making such AI applications more autonomous and intelligent. Common XAI techniques for this purpose include fuzzy inference rules, decision rules (or trees), random forests, and locally interpretable model-agnostic explanations (LIME).

Chapter 4, XAmI Applications to Location-aware Services, is devoted to location-aware (or location-based) services (LASs) that are probably the most prevalent application of ambient intelligence (AmI). This chapter first summarizes the applications of artificial intelligence (AI) in LASs. However, some AI applications in LASs are difficult to understand or communicate with mobile users, so explainable artificial intelligence (XAI) techniques must be applied to enhance the understandability of such AI applications. To this end, some XAI techniques for LASs have been introduced. Subsequently, various types of interpretations of LASs are explained through examples. In addition, the priorities and impacts of criteria for choosing suitable service locations are also distinguished. Furthermore, to enhance the interpretability of the recommendation process and result for users, visualization XAI methods tailored for LASs are also reviewed. This section concludes with a discussion of how to interpret AI-based optimization in LASs.

Chapter 5, XAI Applications to Telemedicine and Telecare, discusses the application of XAI to telemedicine and telecare which are another important application of ambient intelligence (AmI). This chapter first summarizes the applications of artificial intelligence (AI) in telemedicine and telecare. Since some of these AI applications are difficult to understand or communicate with patients, various explainable artificial intelligence (XAI) techniques have been applied, such as shape-added explanation value (SHAP) analysis and locally interpretable model-agnostic explanation (LIME) to overcome such difficulties. Telemedicine services for type-II diabetes diagnosis are taken as an example to illustrate such applications. Several issues with existing XAI applications in telemedicine and telecare are then discussed. It is worth noting that after SHAP analysis, some important attributes may be difficult to measure by patients themselves, which affects the utility of telemedicine or healthcare applications.

References

1. K. Ducatel, M. Bogdanowicz, F. Scapolo, J. Leijten, J.C. Burgelman, *Scenarios for Ambient Intelligence in 2010* (Office for Official Publications of the European Communities, Luxembourg, 2001)
2. T.C.T. Chen, M.C. Chiu, Mining the preferences of patients for ubiquitous clinic recommendation. Health Care Manag. Sci. **23**, 173–184 (2020)
3. F. Sadri, Ambient intelligence: a survey. ACM Comput. Surv. **43**(4), 36 (2011)
4. M.C. Chiu, T. Chen, Assessing mobile and smart technology applications for active and healthy aging using a fuzzy collaborative intelligence approach. Cogn. Comput. **13**, 431–446 (2021)
5. T.C.T. Chen, Y.C. Wang, An incremental learning and integer-nonlinear programming approach to mining users' unknown preferences for ubiquitous hotel recommendation. J. Ambient. Intell. Humaniz. Comput. **10**, 2771–2780 (2019)
6. C. Stephanidis, M. Antona, S. Ntoa, in *Handbook of Human Factors and Ergonomics*. Human Factors in Ambient Intelligence Environments (2021), pp. 1058–1084
7. D. Aggarwal, T. Hoang, B. Ploderer, F. Vetere, R.A. Khot, M. Bradford, in *Proceedings of the 32nd Australian Conference on Human-Computer Interaction*. Lessons Learnt from Designing a Smart Clothing Telehealth System for Hospital Use (2020), pp. 355–367
8. T.C.T. Chen, in *Sustainable Smart Healthcare: Lessons Learned from the COVID-19 Pandemic*. Smart Technology Applications in Healthcare Before, During, and After the COVID-19 Pandemic (2023), pp. 19–37
9. N. Ju, K.H. Lee, Consumer resistance to innovation: smart clothing. Fashion Text. **7**, 1–19 (2020)
10. H.C. Wu, T. Chen, C.H. Huang, A piecewise linear FGM approach for efficient and accurate FAHP analysis: smart backpack design as an example. Mathematics **8**(8), 1319 (2020)
11. Fortunebusinessinsights.com, The global smart home market size was valued at \$80.21 billion in 2022 & is projected to grow from \$93.98 billion in 2023 to \$338.28 billion by 2030 (2022). https://www.fortunebusinessinsights.com/industry-reports/smart-home-market-101900
12. T. Chen, Y.C. Wang, Recommending suitable smart technology applications to support mobile healthcare after the COVID-19 pandemic using a fuzzy approach. Healthcare **9**(11), 1461 (2021)
13. D.J. Cook, M. Youngblood, S.K. Das, A multi-agent approach to controlling a smart environment. Lecture Notes Artif. Intell. **4008**, 165–206 (2006)
14. T. Chen, Enhancing the performance of a ubiquitous location-aware service system using a fuzzy collaborative problem solving strategy. Comput. Ind. Eng. **87**, 296–307 (2015)
15. T.C.T. Chen, in *Production Planning and Control in Semiconductor Manufacturing: Big Data Analytics and Industry 4.0 Applications*. Industry 4.0 for Semiconductor Manufacturing (2023), pp. 21–40
16. M.T. Wang, C.C. Yang, Concept design from random algorithms for design sketching. J. Ambient. Intell. Humaniz. Comput. **6**, 3–11 (2015)
17. A.M. Otebolaku, M.T. Andrade, Context-aware media recommendations for smart devices. J. Ambient. Intell. Humaniz. Comput. **6**, 13–36 (2015)
18. T.C.T. Chen, in *Production Planning and Control in Semiconductor Manufacturing: Big Data Analytics and Industry 4.0 Applications*. Cycle Time Prediction and Output Projection (2023), pp. 41–62
19. A. Van den Oord, S. Dieleman, B. Schrauwen, Deep content-based music recommendation. Adv. Neural. Inf. Process. Syst. **26**, 1–9 (2013)
20. Y.C. Wang, T.C.T. Chen, M.C. Chiu, A systematic approach to enhance the explainability of artificial intelligence in healthcare with application to diagnosis of diabetes. Healthcare Anal. **3**, 100183 (2023)
21. T. Chen, Ubiquitous multicriteria clinic recommendation system. J. Med. Syst. **40**, 1–11 (2016)

22. J. Malczewski, X. Liu, Local ordered weighted averaging in GIS-based multicriteria analysis. Ann. GIS **20**(2), 117–129 (2014)
23. T.C.T. Chen, in *Explainable Artificial Intelligence (XAI) in Manufacturing: Methodology, Tools, and Applications*. Applications of XAI for Decision Making in Manufacturing (2023), pp. 51–81
24. W. Campos, A. Martinez, W. Sanchez, H. Estrada, N.A. Castro-Sánchez, D. Mujica, A systematic review of proposals for the social integration of elderly people using ambient intelligence and social networking sites. Cogn. Comput. **8**, 529–542 (2016)
25. E. Pisula, Z. Kossakowska, Sense of coherence and coping with stress among mothers and fathers of children with autism. J. Autism Dev. Disord. **40**(12), 1485–1494 (2010)
26. T.-C.T. Chen, Y.-C. Wang, in *Artificial Intelligence and Lean Manufacturing*. AI Applications to Kaizen Management (2022), pp. 37–52
27. H.C. Wu, T.C.T. Chen, M.C. Chiu, Assessing the sustainability of smart healthcare applications using a multi-perspective fuzzy comprehensive evaluation approach. Digital Health **9**, 20552076231203904 (2023)
28. T.C.T. Chen, C.W. Lin, An FGM decomposition-based fuzzy MCDM method for selecting smart technology applications to support mobile health care during and after the COVID-19 pandemic. Appl. Soft Comput. **121**, 108758 (2022)
29. H. Gao J. Tang X. Hu, H. Liu, in *Proceedings of the 7th ACM Conference on Recommender Systems*. Exploring Temporal Effects for Location Recommendation on Location-Based Social Networks (2013), pp. 93–100
30. T.C.T. Chen, T.C. Chang, Y.C. Wang, Improving people's health by burning low-pollution coal to improve air quality for thermal power generation. Digital Health **9**, 20552076231185280 (2023)
31. M. Allamanis, S. Scellato, C. Mascolo, in *Proceedings of the 2012 Internet Measurement Conference*. Evolution of a Location-Based Online Social Network: Analysis and Models (2012), pp. 145–158
32. T. Chen, K. Honda, Solving data preprocessing problems in existing location-aware systems. J. Ambient. Intell. Humaniz. Comput. **9**(2), 253–260 (2018)
33. N. Thakur, C.Y. Han, An ambient intelligence-based human behavior monitoring framework for ubiquitous environments. Information **12**(2), 81 (2021)
34. Y.C. Wang, T.C.T. Chen, Analyzing the impact of COVID-19 vaccination requirements on travelers' selection of hotels using a fuzzy multi-criteria decision-making approach. Healthcare Anal. **2**, 100064 (2022)
35. D. Buhalis, Technology in tourism-from information communication technologies to eTourism and smart tourism towards ambient intelligence tourism: a perspective article. Tourism Rev. **75**(1), 267–272 (2020)
36. H.C. Wu, Y.C. Lin, T.C.T. Chen, Leisure agricultural park selection for traveler groups amid the COVID-19 pandemic. Agriculture **12**(1), 111 (2022)
37. A. Costa, J.A. Rincon, C. Carrascosa, V. Julian, P. Novais, Emotions detection on an ambient intelligent system using wearable devices. Futur. Gener. Comput. Syst. **92**, 479–489 (2019)
38. M.C. Chiu, T.C.T. Chen, Assessing sustainable effectiveness of the adjustment mechanism of a ubiquitous clinic recommendation system. Health Care Manag. Sci. **23**, 239–248 (2020)
39. T. Chen, Y.C. Wang, Interval fuzzy number-based approach for modeling an uncertain fuzzy yield learning process. J. Ambient. Intell. Humaniz. Comput. **11**, 1213–1223 (2020)
40. X. Wan, T. Okamoto, Utilizing learning process to improve recommender system for group learning support. Neural Comput. Appl. **20**, 611–621 (2011)
41. T.C.T. Chen, in *Production Planning and Control in Semiconductor Manufacturing: Big Data Analytics and Industry 4.0 Applications*. Defect Pattern Analysis, Yield Learning Modeling, and Yield Prediction (2023), pp. 63–76
42. Y.C. Wang, T.C.T. Chen, H.C. Wu, A novel auto-weighting deep-learning fuzzy collaborative intelligence approach. Decis. Anal. J. **6**, 100186 (2023)
43. T. Chen, C.W. Lin, Smart and automation technologies for ensuring the long-term operation of a factory amid the COVID-19 pandemic: an evolving fuzzy assessment approach. Int. J. Adv. Manuf. Technol. **111**, 3545–3558 (2020)

44. T. Chen, Evaluating the sustainability of a smart technology application to mobile health care—the FGM-ACO-FWA approach. Compl. Intell. Syst. **6**, 109–121 (2020)
45. Y.C. Wang, T. Chen, Y.C. Lin, A collaborative and ubiquitous system for fabricating dental parts using 3D printing technologies. Healthcare **7**(3), 103 (2019)
46. H.C. Wu, T.C.T. Chen, C.H. Huang, Y.C. Shih, Comparing built-in power banks for a smart backpack design using an auto-weighting fuzzy-weighted-intersection FAHP approach. Mathematics **8**(10), 1759 (2020)
47. C. Röcker, Ambient intelligence in the production and retail sector: Emerging opportunities and potential pitfalls. Int. J. Inf. Commun. Eng. **3**(5), 592–603 (2009)
48. T. Chen, H.R. Tsai, Application of industrial engineering concepts and techniques to ambient intelligence: a case study. J. Ambient. Intell. Humaniz. Comput. **9**, 215–223 (2018)
49. M.Á. Sánchez-Cifo, F. Montero, M.T. Lopez, A methodology for emotional intelligence testing in elderly people with low-cost EEG and PPG devices. J. Ambient. Intell. Humaniz. Comput. **14**(3), 2351–2367 (2023)
50. H.C. Wu, Y.C. Wang, T.C.T. Chen, Assessing and comparing COVID-19 intervention strategies using a varying partial consensus fuzzy collaborative intelligence approach. Mathematics **8**(10), 1725 (2020)
51. R.J. Aldrich, D. Richterova, in *Secrecy in European Politics*. Ambient Accountability: Intelligence Services in Europe and the Decline of State Secrecy (2020), pp. 179–200
52. T. Chen, M.C. Chiu, A fuzzy collaborative intelligence approach to group decision-making: a case study of post-COVID-19 restaurant transformation. Cogn. Comput. **14**(2), 531–546 (2022)
53. Y.-C. Lin, T. Chen, An intelligent system for assisting personalized COVID-19 vaccination location selection: Taiwan as an example. Digital Health **8**, 20552076221109064 (2022)
54. H. Kim, S. Jung, G. Ryu, A study on the restaurant recommendation service app based on AI chatbot using personalization information. Int. J. Adv. Culture Technol. **8**(4), 263–270 (2020)
55. T.C.T. Chen, in *Sustainable Smart Healthcare: Lessons Learned from the COVID-19 Pandemic*. Sustainable Smart Healthcare Applications: Lessons Learned from the COVID-19 Pandemic (2023), pp. 65–92
56. D. Magliocchetti, M. Gielow, F. De Vigili, G. Conti, R. De Amicis, A personal mobility assistant based on ambient intelligence to promote sustainable travel choices. Proc. Comput. Sci. **5**, 892–899 (2011)
57. T.C.T. Chen, in *Sustainable Smart Healthcare: Lessons Learned from the COVID-19 Pandemic*. Smart Healthcare (2023), pp. 1–18
58. Y.C. Wang, T. Chen, M.-C. Chiu, An improved explainable artificial intelligence tool in healthcare for hospital recommendation. Healthcare Anal. **3**, 100147 (2023)
59. T.C.T. Chen, H.C. Wu, A partial-consensus and unequal-authority fuzzy collaborative intelligence approach for assessing robotic applications amid the COVID-19 pandemic. Soft. Comput. **27**(22), 16493–16509 (2023)
60. M. Ziefle, C. Röcker, W. Wilkowska, K. Kasugai, L. Klack, C. Möllering, S. Beul, in *E-Health, Assistive Technologies and Applications for Assisted Living: Challenges and Solutions*. A Multi-Disciplinary Approach to Ambient Assisted Living (2011), pp. 76–93
61. Y.C. Lin, Y.C. Wang, T.C.T. Chen, H.F. Lin, Evaluating the suitability of a smart technology application for fall detection using a fuzzy collaborative intelligence approach. Mathematics **7**(11), 1097 (2019)
62. T.C.T. Chen, in *Sustainable Smart Healthcare: Lessons Learned from the COVID-19 Pandemic*. Evaluating the Sustainability of a Smart Healthcare Application (2023), pp. 39–63
63. T. Chen, Y.C. Wang, M.C. Chiu, A type-II fuzzy collaborative forecasting approach for productivity forecasting under an uncertainty environment. J. Ambient. Intell. Humaniz. Comput. **12**, 2751–2763 (2021)
64. Y. Ghadi, B. Mouazma, M. Gochoo, A. Suliman, S. Tamara, A. Jalal, J. Park, Improving the ambient intelligence living using deep learning classifier. Comput. Mater. Contin. **73**(1), 1037–1053 (2022)

65. T. Chen, Y.C. Wang, A modified random forest incremental interpretation method for explaining artificial and deep neural networks in cycle time prediction. Decis. Anal. J. **7**, 100226 (2023)
66. J.C. Kim, K. Chung, Neural-network based adaptive context prediction model for ambient intelligence. J. Ambient. Intell. Humaniz. Comput. **11**, 1451–1458 (2020)
67. T.C.T. Chen, Y.C. Lin, Fuzzified deep neural network ensemble approach for estimating cycle time range. Appl. Soft Comput. **130**, 109697 (2022)
68. H. Tabatabaee Malazi, M. Davari, Combining emerging patterns with random forest for complex activity recognition in smart homes. Appl. Intell. **48**(2), 315–330 (2018)
69. T. Chen, Y.C. Wang, A two-stage explainable artificial intelligence approach for classification-based job cycle time prediction. Int. J. Adv. Manuf. Technol. **123**(5–6), 2031–2042 (2022)
70. F. Doctor, H. Hagras, V. Callaghan, A type-2 fuzzy embedded agent to realise ambient intelligence in ubiquitous computing environments. Inf. Sci. **171**(4), 309–334 (2005)
71. T.-C.T. Chen, Type-II fuzzy collaborative intelligence for assessing cloud manufacturing technology applications. Rob. Comput. Integ. Manuf. **78**, 102399 (2022)
72. Y. Geng, J. Chen, R. Fu, G. Bao, K. Pahlavan, Enlighten wearable physiological monitoring systems: on-body rf characteristics based human motion classification using a support vector machine. IEEE Trans. Mob. Comput. **15**(3), 656–671 (2015)
73. T.C.T. Chen, Y.C. Wang, in *Artificial Intelligence and Lean Manufacturing*. AI Applications to Shop Floor Management in Lean Manufacturing (2022), pp. 75–90
74. S.A. Changazi, A.D. Bakhshi, M. Yousaf, M.H. Islam, S.M. Mohsin, S.S. Band, A. Alsufyani, S. Bourouis, GA-based geometrically optimized topology robustness to improve ambient intelligence for future internet of things. Comput. Commun. **193**, 109–117 (2022)
75. T.C.T. Chen, C.W. Lin, M.C. Chiu, Optimizing 3D printing facility selection for ubiquitous manufacturing using an evolving fuzzy big data analytics approach. Int. J. Adv. Manuf. Technol. **127**, 4111–4121 (2023)
76. F.N.A. Baharudin, N.A. Ab. Aziz, M.R. Abdul Malek, Z. Ibrahim, in *RiTA 2020: Proceedings of the 8th International Conference on Robot Intelligence Technology and Applications*. Optimization of User Comfort Index for Ambient Intelligence Using Dynamic Inertia Weight Artificial Bees Colony Optimization Algorithm (2021), pp. 351–363
77. H. Hagras, V. Callaghan, M. Colley, G. Clarke, A. Pounds-Cornish, H. Duman, Creating an ambient-intelligence environment using embedded agents. IEEE Intell. Syst. **19**(6), 12–20 (2004)
78. T.C.T. Chen, Y.C. Wang, Fuzzy dynamic-prioritization agent-based system for forecasting job cycle time in a wafer fabrication plant. Compl. Intell. Syst. **7**, 2141–2154 (2021)
79. M. McNamara, Explainable AI: what is it? How does it work? And what role does data play? (2022). https://www.netapp.com/blog/explainable-ai/
80. D. Kumar, A. Wong, G.W. Taylor, in *Proceedings of the IEEE Conference on Computer Vision and Pattern Recognition Workshops*. Explaining the Unexplained: A Class-Enhanced Attentive Response (Clear) Approach to Understanding Deep Neural Networks (2017), pp. 36–44
81. D. Gunning, D. Aha, DARPA's explainable artificial intelligence (XAI) program. AI Mag. **40**(2), 44–58 (2019)
82. T. Chen, M.-C. Chiu, Evaluating the sustainability of a smart technology application in healthcare after the COVID-19 pandemic: a hybridizing subjective and objective fuzzy group decision-making approach with XAI. Digital Health **8**, 20552076221136380 (2022)
83. Y.C. Wang, T. Chen, New XAI tools for selecting suitable 3D printing facilities in ubiquitous manufacturing. Compl. Intell. Syst. **9**, 6813–6829 (2023)
84. T.C.T. Chen, Enhancing the sustainability of smart healthcare applications with XAI. in *Sustainable Smart Healthcare: Lessons Learned from the COVID-19 Pandemic* (2023), pp. 93–100
85. J. Cassens, R. Wegener, in *European Conference on Ambient Intelligence*. Ambient Explanations: Ambient Intelligence and Explainable AI (2019), pp. 370–376

86. U. Kamath, J. Liu, *Explainable Artificial Intelligence: An Introduction to Interpretable Machine Learning* (Springer, 2021)
87. T.C.T. Chen, in *Explainable Artificial Intelligence (XAI) in Manufacturing: Methodology, Tools, and Applications*. Applications of XAI to Job Sequencing and Scheduling in Manufacturing (2023), pp. 83–105
88. Y.C. Wang, T. Chen, Adapted techniques of explainable artificial intelligence for explaining genetic algorithms on the example of job scheduling. Exp. Syst. Appl. 237(A), 121369 (2024)
89. T.C.T. Chen, H.C. Wu, K.W. Hsu, A fuzzy analytic hierarchy process-enhanced fuzzy geometric mean-fuzzy technique for order preference by similarity to ideal solution approach for suitable hotel recommendation amid the COVID-19 pandemic. Digital Health **8**, 20552076221084456 (2022)
90. A. Schmidt, in *Ambient Intelligence*. Interactive Context-Aware Systems Interacting with Ambient Intelligence (2005), pp. 159–178
91. M. Hörwick, K.H. Siedersberger, in *2010 IEEE Intelligent Vehicles Symposium*. Strategy and Architecture of a Safety Concept for Fully Automatic and Autonomous Driving Assistance Systems (2010), pp. 955–960
92. T.C.T. Chen, in *Explainable Artificial Intelligence (XAI) in Manufacturing: Methodology, Tools, and Applications*. Explainable Artificial Intelligence (XAI) in Manufacturing (2023), pp. 1–11
93. M.R. Zafar, N. Khan, Deterministic local interpretable model-agnostic explanations for stable explainability. Mach. Learn. Knowl. Extract. 3(3), 525–541 (2021)
94. K. Mouloudel, A. Chibani, H. Abdelkawy, Y. Amirat, in *2022 IEEE 18th International Conference on Automation Science and Engineering*. Hybrid Approach for Anticipating Human Activities in Ambient Intelligence Environments (2022), pp. 2006–2011
95. Y.-C. Lin, T. Chen, Type-II fuzzy approach with explainable artificial intelligence for nature-based leisure travel destination selection amid the COVID-19 pandemic. Digital Health **8**, 20552076221106320 (2022)
96. T.C.T. Chen, in *Advances in Fuzzy Group Decision Making*. Consensus Measurement and Enhancement (2021), pp. 55–72
97. A. Bertrand, R. Belloum, J.R. Eagan, W. Maxwell, in *Proceedings of the 2022 AAAI/ACM Conference on AI, Ethics, and Society*. How Cognitive Biases Affect XAI-Assisted Decision-Making: A Systematic Review (2022), pp. 78–91
98. T.C.T. Chen, C.W. Lin, Y.C. Lin, A fuzzy collaborative forecasting approach based on XAI applications for cycle time range estimation. Appl. Soft Comput. **151**, 111122 (2024)
99. J.R. Rehse, N. Mehdiyev, P. Fettke, Towards explainable process predictions for industry 4.0 in the dfki-smart-lego-factory. KI-Künstliche Intelligenz **33**, 181–187 (2019)
100. H. Mankodiya, D. Jadav, R. Gupta, S. Tanwar, A. Alharbi, A. Tolba et al., XAI-fall: Explainable AI for fall detection on wearable devices using sequence models and XAI techniques. Mathematics **10**(12), 1990 (2022)
101. V.K. Venugopal, R. Takhar, S. Gupta, V. Mahajan, Clinical explainability failure (CEF) & explainability failure ratio (EFR)—changing the way we validate classification algorithms. J. Med. Syst. **46**(4), 1–5 (2022)
102. N. Barakat, A.P. Bradley, M.N.H. Barakat, Intelligible support vector machines for diagnosis of diabetes mellitus. IEEE Trans. Inf. Technol. Biomed. **14**(4), 1114–1120 (2010)
103. P. Nagaraj, V. Muneeswaran, A. Dharanidharan, K. Balananthanan, M. Arunkumar, C. Rajkumar, in *2022 International Conference on Sustainable Computing and Data Communication Systems*. A Prediction and Recommendation System for Diabetes Mellitus Using XAI-Based Lime Explainer (2022), pp. 1472–1478
104. T.C.T. Chen, in *Explainable Artificial Intelligence (XAI) in Manufacturing: Methodology, Tools, and Applications*. Applications of XAI for Forecasting in the Manufacturing Domain (2023), pp. 13–50

Chapter 2
Explainable Artificial Intelligence (XAI) with Applications

Abstract This chapter begins by defining explainable artificial intelligence (XAI). The explainabilities of existing ML models are then compared, showing the need for XAI applications to improve the explainabilities of some ML models. To this end, XAI techniques and tools for interpreting and enhancing artificial intelligence applications, especially in the field of ambient intelligence (AmI), are discussed. Subsequently, the requirements for trustable AI and XAI are listed. Various classifications of existing XAI methods are then performed to meet these requirements. A literature analysis was also conducted on the application of XAI in various fields, showing that services, medicine, and education are the most common application fields of XAI. Finally, several types of explanations are introduced. XAI techniques for feature importance evaluation are also described.

Keyword Artificial intelligence · Explainable artificial intelligence · Classification · Explanation

2.1 Explainable Artificial Intelligence (XAI)

Artificial intelligence (AI) is a set of technologies that enable computers to imitate human behavior. The computing speed, storage capacity, reliability, and interconnectivity of computers combined with human reasoning patterns give AI the ability to solve complex and large-scale problems. So far, AI applications have penetrated into every aspect of our daily lives [1]. However, the applied AI technologies are becoming increasingly complex, limiting the interpretability and credibility of related applications [2]. Explainable artificial intelligence (XAI) is to enhance the practicality of an existing AI technology by explaining its reasoning process and/or result [3–4].

According to the Defense Advanced Research Projects Agency (DARPA), XAI is designed to produce more interpretable machine learning (ML) models while maintaining high levels of the learning performance (predictive accuracy). XAI enables humans to understand, appropriately trust, and effectively manage these AI applications or their agents [4]. In addition, the General Data Protection Regulation (GDPR)

© The Author(s), under exclusive license to Springer Nature Switzerland AG 2024   23
T.-C. T. Chen, *Explainable Ambient Intelligence (XAmI)*,
SpringerBriefs in Applied Sciences and Technology,
https://doi.org/10.1007/978-3-031-54935-9_2

implemented in European countries states that customers have the right to interpret decisions made through automated systems [5]. All in all, XAI enhances the practicality of an existing AI technology by explaining its reasoning process and/or results. XAI also aims to improve the effectiveness of existing AI technologies by incorporating easy-to-interpret visual features such as heatmaps [6], decision (or regression) rules [7], decision trees (DTs) [8], and scatter plots [9] to help diagnose its reasoning mechanism.

2.2 Explainability of ML Models

Explainability has four aspects [10–11]:

- Understandability (or intelligibility): The model is understandable and does not require any details or explanation of its internal algorithms.
- Comprehensibility: The model can represent and convey the knowledge it has learned.
- Interpretability (or explainability): The structure of the model can be described in a way that is easy for humans to understand.
- Transparency: The internal structure (structural transparency) and algorithm (algorithmic transparency) by which it makes predictions is understandable.

Based on the four criteria, ML models are divided into two categories [12]:

- Highly explainable AI methods, white boxes, crystal-clear models: ensemble methods [13], DTs [8], fuzzy logic [14], case-based reasoning (CBR) [15], expert systems [16], Bayesian networks [17], sparse linear models [18], etc.
- Less explainable AI methods, black boxes: artificial neural networks (ANNs) [15], deep learning [19], random forests (RFs) [19], advanced fuzzy logic [9], support vector machines (SVMs) [20], bio-inspired algorithms (genetic algorithm (GA) [21], artificial bee colony (ABC) [22], particle swarm optimization (PSO) [23], etc.), agent-based systems, etc.

2.3 XAI for Explaining and Enhancing AI Applications in Ambient Intelligence (AmI)

Decision and regression rules have been widely used to explain the inference mechanisms of deep neural networks (DNNs) [8, 24–25]. Attention-based DNNs [26–27] combine DNNs with heatmaps. In other words, heatmaps are used to show the parts of an image that DNNs emphasize when classifying or identifying patterns [28–29].

The concept of locally interpretable model-agnostic explanation (LIME) is to use machine learning models to explain classification or regression results by identifying key features/predictors and fitting simple and locally interpretable models [30–31]. In LIME, synthetic data is used to avoid the influence of extreme cases, thereby improving the prediction performance for test data. For example, a RF can be constructed to approximate a DNN [19, 32–33], in which multiple decision rules are listed, and then unreasonable decision rules are deleted based on domain knowledge, thereby improving the rationality and effectiveness of applying to new cases [34–35].

Chen [3] believed that the domains where XAI is most commonly applied include medical care, services, education, manufacturing, and healthcare, which implied the great potential of ambient intelligence (AmI) (see Fig. 2.1). First of all, telemedicine [36–37], as an innovative medical treatment method, can selectively apply XAI technique and tools in this domain. The same goes for smart homes. In addition, location-aware services (LAS) [38] are popular applications of AmI and belong to the fields of services (such as hotel recommendation services or apps), education (such as healthcare information apps), and healthcare, so are smart factories [39–40].

AI applications in different fields of AmI have different focuses and different goals to be achieved [41–42]. For example, in telemedicine, AI applications strive for an acceptable performance in every case. Therefore, local interpretation is crucial in this field and needs to be optimized. As in other domains or fields of AmI, the number of applications of XAI in telemedicine is still small [37, 43–44], but there have been

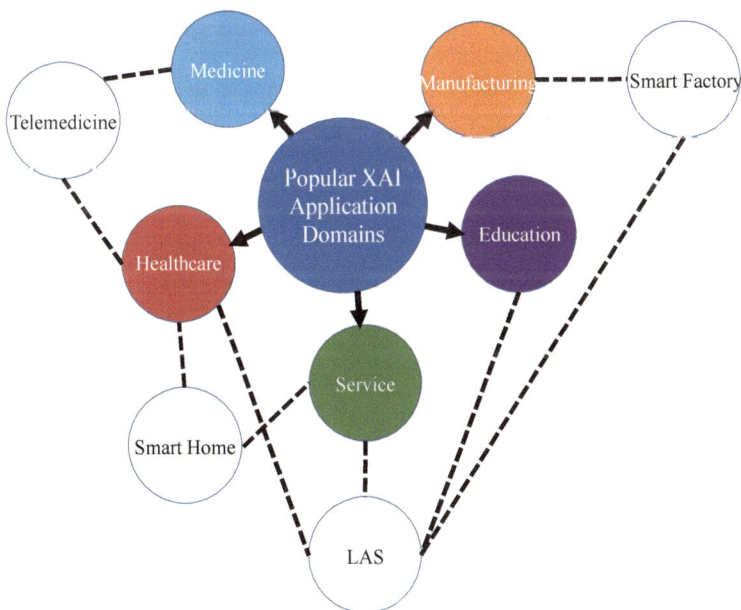

Fig. 2.1 Great potential of XAI applications in the fields of AmI

some comments on possible applications of XAI in this field [45–46]. While this is strange, it reaffirms the huge potential of XAI for telemedicine. In contrast, in LAS, it is challenging for AI applications to satisfy the needs of all users [47]. Therefore, the failure in one case can be compensated by the success in another. AI applications in this field usually pursue the optimization of the average performance.

2.4 Requirements for Trustable AI and XAI

The requirements for trustworthy AI and XAI are as follows (see Fig. 2.2) [10]:

- Informativeness: XAI gives us information about the goals our AI models are trying to achieve, so we can evaluate whether those goals are inconsistent with our intentions, misleading, or counterproductive.
- Credibility: AI algorithms should be relevant, easy to understand, and not prone to misinformation.
- Fairness: AI applications need to treat users or actions fairly, without any favoritism or discrimination.
- Transparency: AI model and algorithm transparency help us understand how specific decisions are made. The applications of XAI techniques must facilitate this [48].
- Cause and Effect: XAI can be used to explore cause-and-effect relationships [49].
- Transferability: Transfer learning is the concept that a model trained on one task can be generalized and used as a starting point for other tasks. The applications of XAI techniques must facilitate this.
- Reliability: AI models make the same decision in the same situation. The applications of XAI techniques must ensure this.

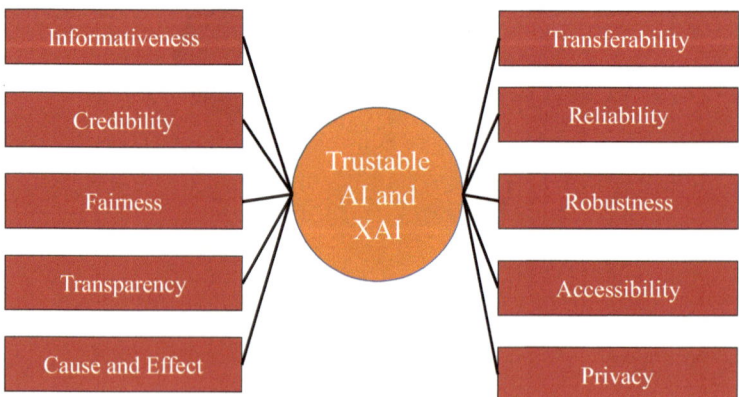

Fig. 2.2 Requirements for trustworthy AI and XAI

- Robustness: AI models make similar decisions in similar situations. The applications of XAI techniques must ensure this [50].
- Accessibility: Non-technical people can access or use AI applications without any difficulty. The applications of XAI techniques must ensure this.
- Privacy: Regulators or governments must be able to easily assess whether an AI application's encrypted representation or algorithm violates privacy [51].

2.5 Classification of XAI Methods

XAI methods can be classified in a variety of ways [10]. For example, considering the time point of application, XAI methods can be divided into

- Pre-model methods: Pre-model methods are independent of the model in that they only apply to the data. Box (and whisker) plots (Fig. 2.3), distribution plots (Fig. 2.4), heatmaps (Fig. 2.5), and violin plots (Fig. 2.6) are prevalent XAI methods for pre-model data analysis.
- Intrinsic methods: Intrinsic methods refer to self-explanatory models (DTs, generalized linear, logistic, and clustering models) that exploit internal structures to provide natural interpretability [52–53].
- Post hoc methods: They explain the global or local behavior of a model by solving the relationship between input samples and their predictions, without requiring knowledge of the internal structure [54].

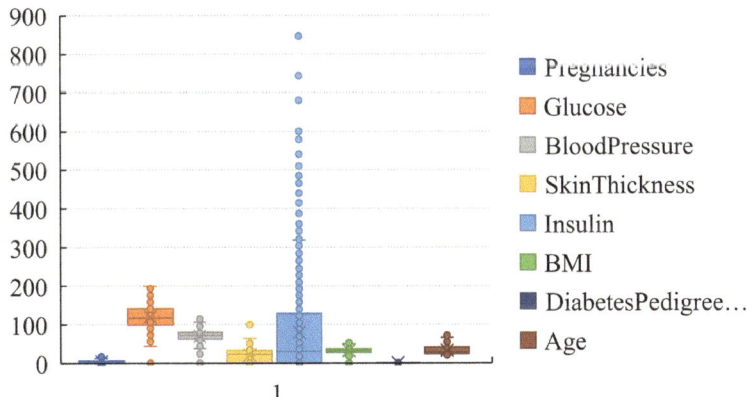

Fig. 2.3 Box-and-whisker plot

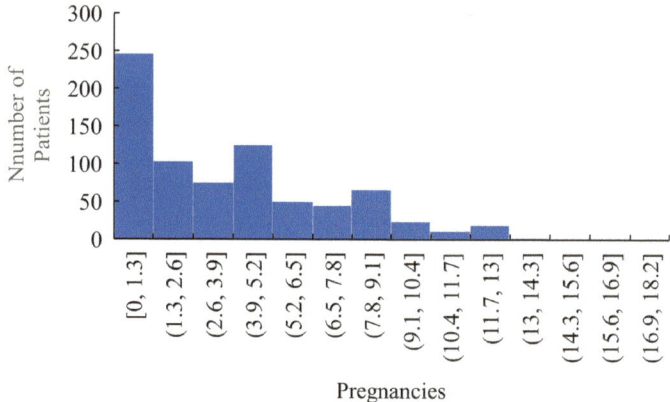

Fig. 2.4 Distribution plot

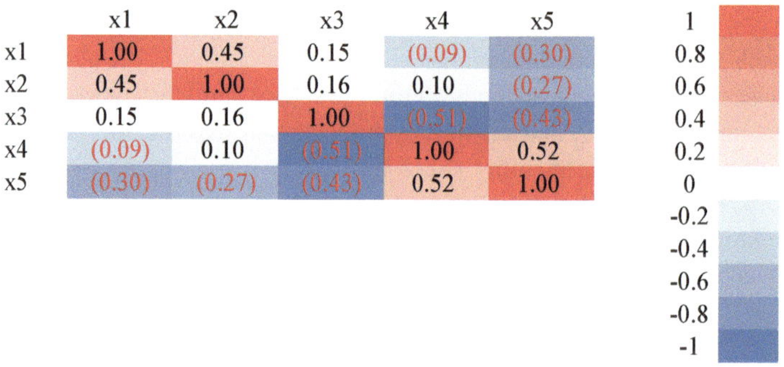

	x1	x2	x3	x4	x5
x1	1.00	0.45	0.15	(0.09)	(0.30)
x2	0.45	1.00	0.16	0.10	(0.27)
x3	0.15	0.16	1.00	(0.51)	(0.43)
x4	(0.09)	0.10	(0.51)	1.00	0.52
x5	(0.30)	(0.27)	(0.43)	0.52	1.00

Fig. 2.5 Heatmap

Fig. 2.6 Violin plot

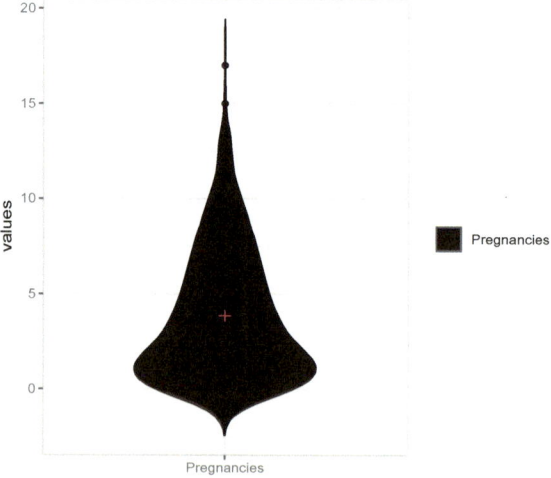

Another classification of XAI methods depends on the tools used and the goals to be achieved:

- XAI techniques and tools for visualizing the operations in AI applications [9, 55].
- XAI techniques and tools for assessing the impact, contribution, or importance of each input to the output [56–57].
- XAI techniques and tools for approximating the relationships between inputs and outputs of AI applications [58–59].

2.6   XAI Applications in Various Domains

According to the survey by [3], the most common application domains of XAI included medicine, services, and education. Compared with this survey, the following points need to be noted:

- The numbers of XAI applications in various fields have shown explosive growth (Fig. 2.7).
- The most common application domains become services, education, and medicine. Reasons for such changes include growing demands for trustworthy AI and XAI in medicine [60–61].

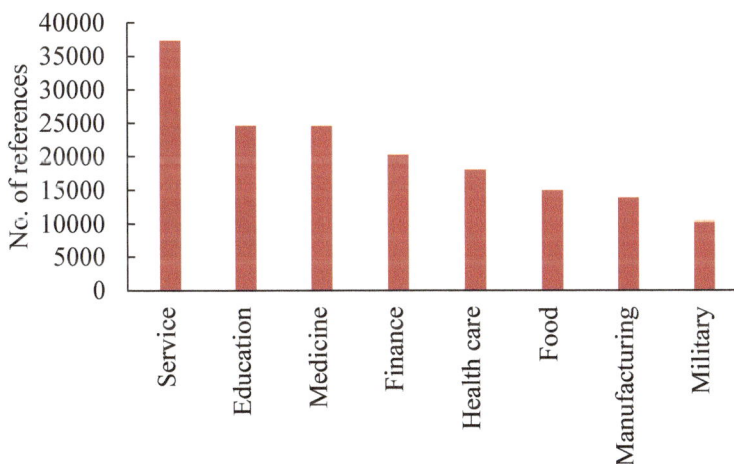

Fig. 2.7 Number of references about XAI applications in various domains from 2010 to 2023 (Data source: Google Scholar)

In sum,

- Appropriate XAI tools will vary depending on the AI methods used, applications, and users (objects to be interpreted).
- Some AI applications require no explanation: For some AI applications, explanation may not be important, and some AI researchers believe that the emphasis on explanation is misplaced, too difficult to achieve, and perhaps unnecessary [4].

2.7   Types of Explanations

There are various types of explanations [10] (see Fig. 2.8):

- Global explanation: How does the model (AI application) work? System diagrams, flow charts, mathematical formulas, pseudocode, and performance indicators are typical examples of global explanations of an AI application.
- Local explanation: Why the model generates the output for a given instance.
- Contrastive explanation (or counterfactual explanation): Why the model generates a certain output rather than another for a given instance. A contrastive explanation helps determine the minimum change in inputs or model parameters required to generate a different output (see Fig. 2.9). Local foil tree method belongs to this type of XAI method.
- What-if explanation: To generate a what-if explanation, a sensitivity analysis or parameter analysis usually needs to be performed.

Fig. 2.8 Types of explanations

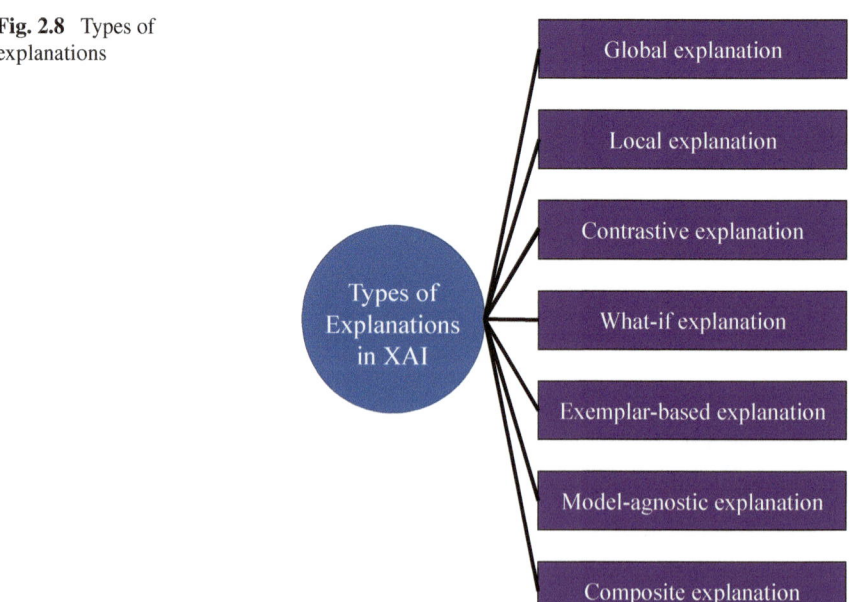

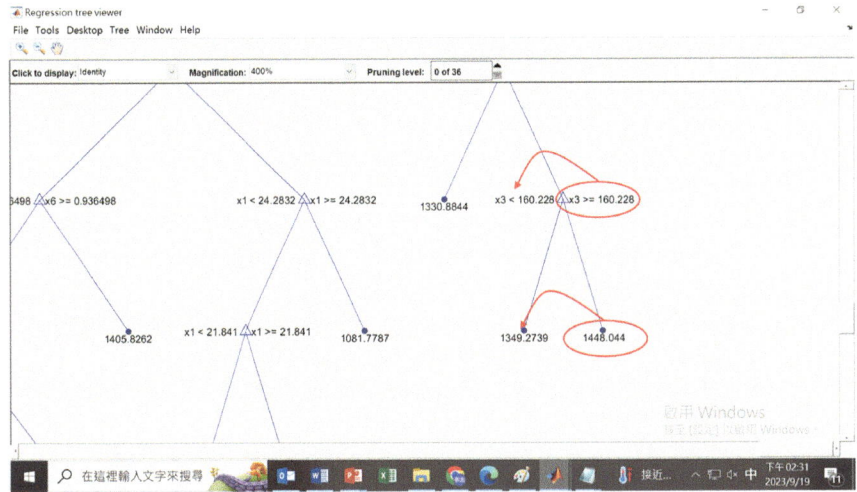

Fig. 2.9 Minimum change in inputs or model parameters required to generate a different output

- Exemplar-based explanation: Users can be presented with similar examples from which the model will generate similar outputs. CBR [15] belongs to this type of XAI method.
- Model-agnostic explanation: A model-agnostic explanation is to explain the calculations required for the AI application that are not based on the parameters of the AI model.
- Composite explanation: When a single explanation cannot accurately explain the reasoning process and results of an AI application, a composite explanation composed of multiple explanations may be needed [19, 33]. Table 2.1 gives an example where an RF of ten decision trees is constructed to assist in diabetes diagnosis. How to organize these explanations to reduce user confusion and improve efficiency is a challenging task. Random forest incremental interpretation (RFII) (see Fig. 2.10) [19] belongs to this type of XAI method. Table 2.2 shows the results of the RFII application for the example in Table 2.1.

Some XAI techniques for generating composite explanations are compared in Table 2.3.

Table 2.1 Composite explanation

Decision rule #	Decision rule[a]
1	If xj8<29.5 and xj2<156 and xj3<37 and xj6>=26.75 then oj=1
2	If xj1<2.5 and xj2<127.5 and xj8<28.5 and xj4<29.5 and xj5<89.5 and xj3<83.5 then oj=0
3	If xj7<0.71 and xj6<38.9 and xj2<99.5 and xj3<84.5 and xj1<11.5 then oj=0
4	If xj2<155.5 and xj7>=0.513 and xj6<32.45 and xj3<87 and 0.5<=xj1<2.5 and xj4>=9 then oj=0
5	If xj5<153.5 and xj2<99.5 and xj3<79 and xj4<40.5 and xj7>=0.298 then oj=0
6	If xj2<123.5 and xj1<3.5 and xj8<28.5 and xj4<34.5 then oj=0
7	If xj2<127.5 and xj1<5.5 and xj7>=0.4955 and xj4<28.5 and xj6>=23.75 and xj8<35 then oj=0
8	If xj2<154.5 and xj7>=0.502 and xj4<34.5 and xj6<32.45 and xj8<31.5 and xj5<175 then oj=0
9	If xj2<105.5 and xj8<23.5 and xj7>=0.419 then oj=0
10	If xj6<29.85 and xj5<119 and xj2<114.5 and xj1<2.5 then oj=0

[a]xj1: number of pregnancies; xj2: blood glucose level; xj3: blood pressure measurement; xj4: thickness of the skin; xj5: insulin level in the blood; xj6: body mass index; xj7: diabetes percentage; xj8: age

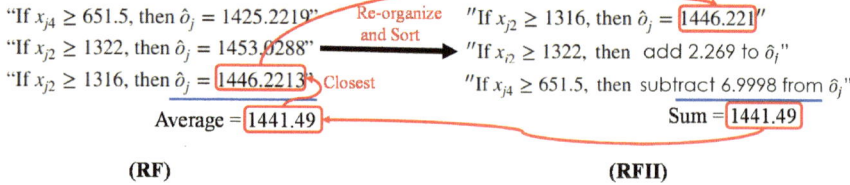

Fig. 2.10 RFII

Table 2.2 RFII application results

RFII rule #	Rule content
1	If xj1<2.5 and xj2<127.5 and xj8<28.5 and xj4<29.5 and xj5<89.5 and xj3<83.5 then oj=0
2	If xj8<29.5 and xj2<156 and xj3<37 and xj6>=26.75 then add 0.1 to oj

Table 2.3 Comparison of some XAI techniques for generating composite explanations

	RF	Gradient boosted decision trees (GBDT)	RF incremental interpretation (RFII) [33]	Modified RFII
Number of decision rules for an example	Many	Many	Many	Many
Each decision rule directly approximates the output	Yes	No	No	No
Attribute importance considered	No	No	No	Yes
First decision rule is the most accurate	No	No	Yes	Yes

2.8 XAI Techniques for Feature Importance Evaluation

XAI techniques and tools for feature importance evaluation are post hoc methods, which include the following:

- Visualization methods: For example, in an ANN, users can observe the network weights of each layer to see how each feature contributes to the output in the next layer (Fig. 2.11). Positive and negative connection weights are displayed in different colors, and the thickness of the line is proportional to the absolute value of the connection weight. However, it is a problem that the difference in the thickness of the lines is not sufficiently noticeable.
- In a Shapley analysis (SHAP), the Sharpley values of attributes, reflecting their importance, can be compared using a force plot or tornado plot. A heatmap is often plotted to illustrate the correlation between attributes and the output.
- Analytic methods: Analytic methods for attribute importance evaluation include correlation analysis, back elimination of regression analysis, contingency table analysis, partial derivation, odd ratio, out-of-bag (OOB) predictor importance, recursive feature elimination (RFE), permutation feature importance (PFI), and SHAP analysis.

RFE is the same as backward elimination regression analysis by searching for a subset of features starting with all features in the training dataset and then removing features until the required number of features remains. The remaining features are considered more important than others. In fact, some machine learning algorithms can be misled by irrelevant input features, resulting in a poor prediction performance on unlearned data.

PFI is defined as the degradation in the model performance when a single feature value is randomly shuffled. This process destroys the relationship between features and the output, so a drop in the model performance indicates how dependent the model is on features. Similar to RFE: RFE removes attributes, while PFI randomizes the attribute's value. The effect is similar.

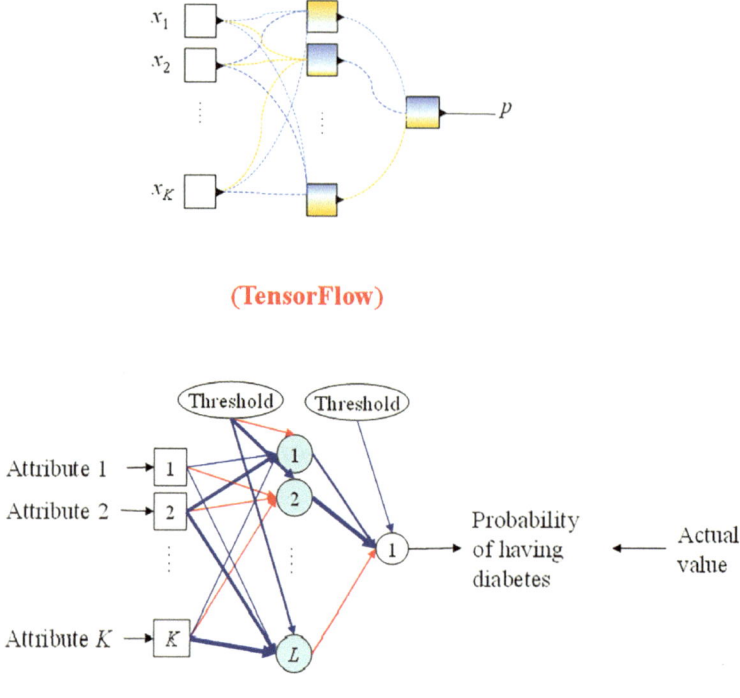

Fig. 2.11 Visualization techniques

SHAP fixes the value of an attribute and randomizes the values of other attributes. The importance of attributes is directly proportional to the model performance. In contrast, PFI randomizes the value of an attribute while fixes the values of other attributes. The importance of an attribute is inversely proportional to the model performance, or the importance of an attribute is directly proportional to the degradation of the model performance.

In decision-making applications of AmI, users often subjectively compare the relative importance of pairs of attributes and then use analytic hierarchy process (AHP) [62–64] or other techniques to derive the absolute importance (or priority) of each attribute from the pairwise comparison results (see Fig. 2.12). The consistency of such comparisons can also be assessed using metrics such as the consistency index (CI) or the consistency ratio (CR). In this situation, it is not necessary to evaluate the importance of attributes using statistical techniques.

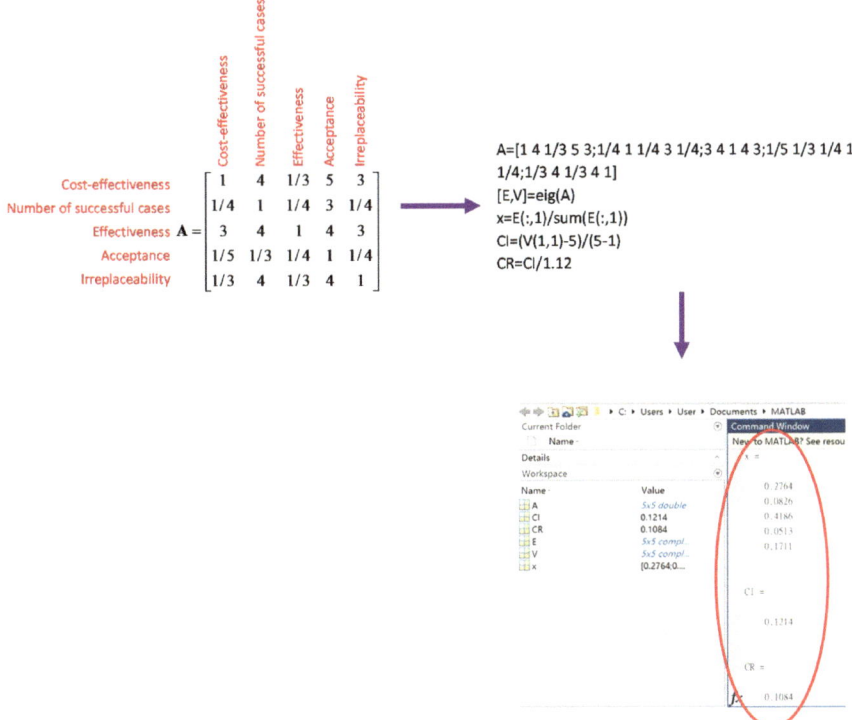

Fig. 2.12 Users subjectively compare and derive the importance of attributes

References

1. T.-C. T. Chen, Y.-C. Wang, in *Artificial Intelligence and Lean Manufacturing*. AI Applications to Kaizen Management, pp. 37–52
2. D. Kumar, A. Wong, G.W. Taylor, in *Proceedings of the IEEE Conference on Computer Vision and Pattern Recognition Workshops*. Explaining the unexplained: A class-enhanced attentive response (clear) approach to understanding deep neural networks (2017), pp. 36–44
3. T.-C.T. Chen, in *Explainable Artificial Intelligence (XAI) in Manufacturing: Methodology, Tools, and Applications*. Explainable Artificial Intelligence (XAI) in Manufacturing (2023), pp. 1–11
4. D. Gunning, D. Aha, DARPA's explainable artificial intelligence (XAI) program. AI Mag. **40**(2), 44–58 (2019)
5. D. Bulgakova, V. Bulgakova, The compliance of facial processing in France with the article 9 paragraph 2 (a)(g) of (EU) general data protection regulation. Regulation **119**, 1 (2016)
6. T.C.T. Chen, in *Production Planning and Control in Semiconductor Manufacturing: Big Data Analytics and Industry 4.0 Applications*. Defect Pattern Analysis, Yield Learning Modeling, and Yield Prediction (2022), pp. 63–76
7. Y.C. Wang, T.C.T. Chen, M.C. Chiu, A systematic approach to enhance the explainability of artificial intelligence in healthcare with application to diagnosis of diabetes. Healthcare Anal. **3**, 100183 (2023)
8. H.-C. Wu, T. Chen, CART–BPN approach for estimating cycle time in wafer fabrication. J. Ambient. Intell. Humaniz. Comput. **6**, 57–67 (2015)

9. Y.-C. Lin, T. Chen, Type-II fuzzy approach with explainable artificial intelligence for nature-based leisure travel destination selection amid the COVID-19 pandemic. Digital Health **8**, 20552076221106320 (2022)
10. U. Kamath, J. Liu, *Explainable Artificial Intelligence: An Introduction to Interpretable Machine Learning* (Springer, 2021)
11. T.C.T. Chen, in *Explainable Artificial Intelligence (XAI) in Manufacturing: Methodology, Tools, and Applications.* Applications of XAI for Forecasting in the Manufacturing Domain (2023), pp. 13–50
12. M. McNamara, Explainable AI: what is it? How does it work? And what role does data play? (2022). https://www.netapp.com/blog/explainable-ai/
13. Q. Xu, V. Sharma, in *Industrial Conference on Data Mining.* Ensemble Sales Forecasting Study in Semiconductor Industry (2017), pp. 31–44
14. T.C.T. Chen, H.C. Wu, K.W. Hsu, A fuzzy analytic hierarchy process-enhanced fuzzy geometric mean-fuzzy technique for order preference by similarity to ideal solution approach for suitable hotel recommendation amid the COVID-19 pandemic. Digital Health **8**, 20552076221084456 (2022)
15. E.M. Kenny, M.T. Keane, in *Twenty-Eighth International Joint Conferences on Artificial Intelligence.* Twin-Systems to Explain Artificial Neural Networks Using Case-Based Reasoning: Comparative Tests of Feature-Weighting Methods in ANN-CBR Twins for XAI (2019), pp. 2708–2715
16. T. Chen, A hybrid fuzzy and neural approach with virtual experts and partial consensus for DRAM price forecasting. Int. J. Innov. Comput. Inf. Control **8**(1), 583–597 (2012)
17. B.G. Marcot, T.D. Penman, Advances in Bayesian network modelling: integration of modelling technologies. Environ Model Softw. **111**, 386–393 (2019)
18. T.A. Davis, S. Rajamanickam, W.M. Sid-Lakhdar, A survey of direct methods for sparse linear systems. Acta Numer. **25**, 383–566 (2016)
19. T. Chen, Y.C. Wang, A modified random forest incremental interpretation method for explaining artificial and deep neural networks in cycle time prediction. Decis. Anal. J. **7**, 100226 (2023)
20. J. Cervantes, F. Garcia-Lamont, L. Rodríguez-Mazahua, A. Lopez, A comprehensive survey on support vector machine classification: applications, challenges and trends. Neurocomputing **408**, 189–215 (2020)
21. T.C.T. Chen, C.W. Lin, M.C. Chiu, Optimizing 3D printing facility selection for ubiquitous manufacturing using an evolving fuzzy big data analytics approach. Int. J. Adv. Manuf. Technol. **127**, 4111–4121 (2023)
22. F.N.A. Baharudin, N.A.A. Aziz, M.R. Abdul Malek, Z. Ibrahim, in *RiTA 2020: Proceedings of the 8th International Conference on Robot Intelligence Technology and Applications.* Optimization of User Comfort Index for Ambient Intelligence Using Dynamic Inertia Weight Artificial Bees Colony Optimization Algorithm (2021), pp. 351–363
23. X. Zhou, H. Ma, J. Gu, H. Chen, W. Deng, Parameter adaptation-based ant colony optimization with dynamic hybrid mechanism. Eng. Appl. Artif. Intell. **114**, 105139 (2022)
24. E. Daglarli, in *Artificial Intelligence Paradigms for Smart Cyber-Physical Systems.* Explainable Artificial Intelligence (xAI) Approaches and Deep Meta-Learning Models for Cyber-Physical Systems (2021), pp. 42–67
25. Y.-C. Wang, T. Chen, T.C. Hsu, A fuzzy deep neural network and simulation approach for enhancing cycle time range estimation precision in wafer fabrication. Decision Anal. **1**, 100010 (2021)
26. E. Choi, M.T. Bahadori, L. Song, W.F. Stewart, J. Sun, in *Proceedings of the 23rd ACM SIGKDD International Conference on Knowledge Discovery and Data Mining.* GRAM: Graph-Based Attention Model for Healthcare Representation Learning (2017), pp. 787–795
27. T.C.T. Chen, in *Explainable Artificial Intelligence (XAI) in Manufacturing: Methodology, Tools, and Applications.* Applications of XAI to Job Sequencing and Scheduling in Manufacturing (2023), pp. 83–105
28. E. Tjoa, H.J. Khok, T. Chouhan, G. Cuntai, Improving deep neural network classification confidence using heatmap-based eXplainable AI (2022). https://doi.org/10.48550/arXiv.2201.000092022

29. T.C.T. Chen, in *Sustainable Smart Healthcare: Lessons Learned from the COVID-19 Pandemic*. Enhancing the Sustainability of Smart Healthcare Applications with XAI (2023), pp. 93–110
30. C. Panigutti, A. Perotti, D. Pedreschi, in *Proceedings of the 2020 Conference on Fairness, Accountability, and Transparency*. Doctor XAI: An Ontology-Based Approach to Black-Box Sequential Data Classification Explanations (2020), pp. 629–639
31. T. Chen, M.-C. Chiu, Evaluating the sustainability of a smart technology application in healthcare after the COVID-19 pandemic: a hybridizing subjective and objective fuzzy group decision-making approach with XAI. Digital Health **8**, 20552076221136380 (2022)
32. B. Gulowaty, M. Woźniak, in *2021 International Joint Conference on Neural Networks*. Extracting Interpretable Decision Tree Ensemble from Random Forest (2021), pp. 1–8
33. T. Chen, Y.C. Wang, A two-stage explainable artificial intelligence approach for classification-based job cycle time prediction. Int. J. Adv. Manuf. Technol. **123**(5), 2031–2042 (2022)
34. M. Rostami, M. Oussalah, A novel explainable COVID-19 diagnosis method by integration of feature selection with random forest. Inf. Med. Unlocked **30**, 100941 (2022)
35. T.C.T. Chen, in *Explainable Artificial Intelligence (XAI) in Manufacturing: Methodology, Tools, and Applications*. Applications of XAI for Decision Making in the Manufacturing Domain (2023), pp. 51–81
36. M.-C. Chiu, T. Chen, A ubiquitous healthcare system of 3D printing facilities for making dentures: application of type-II fuzzy logic. Digital Health **8**, 20552076221092540 (2022)
37. P. Guleria, P. Naga Srinivasu, S. Ahmed, N. Almusallam, F.K. Alarfaj, XAI framework for cardiovascular disease prediction using classification techniques. Electronics **11**(24), 4086 (2022)
38. Y.-C. Lin, T. Chen, An intelligent system for assisting personalized COVID-19 vaccination location selection: Taiwan as an example. Digital Health **8**, 20552076221109064 (2022)
39. Y.-C. Wang, T. Chen, Y.-C. Lin, 3D printer selection for aircraft component manufacturing using a nonlinear FGM and dependency-considered fuzzy VIKOR approach. Aerospace **10**, 591 (2023)
40. T.C.T. Chen, Y.C. Wang, in *Artificial Intelligence and Lean Manufacturing*. AI Applications to Shop Floor Management in Lean Manufacturing (2022), pp. 75–90
41. J.F. Arinez, Q. Chang, R.X. Gao, C. Xu, J. Zhang, Artificial intelligence in advanced manufacturing: current status and future outlook. J. Manuf. Sci. Eng. **142**(11), 110804 (2020)
42. T.C.T. Chen, H.C. Wu, A partial-consensus and unequal-authority fuzzy collaborative intelligence approach for assessing robotic applications amid the COVID-19 pandemic. Soft. Comput. **27**(22), 16493–16509 (2023)
43. M. Lo Giudice, N. Mammone, C. Ieracitano, U. Aguglia, D. Mandic, F.C. Morabito, in *International Conference on Applied Intelligence and Informatics*. Explainable Deep Learning Classification of Respiratory Sound for Telemedicine Applications (2022), pp. 391–403
44. A. Najjar, N. Hosseini-Kivanani, I. Tchappi Haman, Y. Mualla, E. Van der Peijl, D. Karpati, C. Schommer, in *Proceedings of the 10th International Conference on Human-Agent Interaction*. XAI: Using Smart Photobooth for Explaining History of Art (2022), pp. 256–259
45. P. Bhattacharya, M.S. Obaidat, D. Savaliya, S. Sanghavi, S. Tanwar, B. Sadaun, in *International Conference on Computer, Information and Telecommunication Systems*. Metaverse Assisted Telesurgery in Healthcare 5.0: An Interplay of Blockchain and Explainable AI (2022), pp. 1–5
46. R.K. Sheu, M.S. Pardeshi, A survey on medical explainable AI (XAI): recent progress, explainability approach, human interaction and scoring system. Sensors **22**(20), 8068 (2022)
47. T. Chen, Y.C. Wang, A calibrated piecewise-linear FGM approach for travel destination recommendation during the COVID-19 pandemic. Appl. Soft Comput. **109**, 107535 (2021)
48. J. Bunn, Working in contexts for which transparency is important: a recordkeeping view of explainable artificial intelligence (XAI). Rec. Manag. J. **30**(2), 143–153 (2020)
49. T. Chen, Y.-C. Wang, M.-C. Chiu, A type-II fuzzy collaborative forecasting approach for productivity forecasting under an uncertainty environment. J. Ambient. Intell. Humaniz. Comput. **12**, 2751–2763 (2021)
50. A. Artelt, V. Vaquet, R. Velioglu, F. Hinder, J. Brinkrolf, M. Schilling, B. Hammer, in *2021 IEEE Symposium Series on Computational Intelligence*. Evaluating Robustness of Counterfactual Explanations (2021), pp. 1–9

51. H.C. Wu, Y.C. Wang, T.C.T. Chen, Assessing and comparing COVID-19 intervention strategies using a varying partial consensus fuzzy collaborative intelligence approach. Mathematics **8**(10), 1725 (2020)
52. J.X. Mi, X. Jiang, L. Luo, Y. Gao, Toward explainable artificial intelligence: a survey and overview on their intrinsic properties. Neurocomputing **563**, 126919 (2024)
53. Y.C. Wang, T.C.T. Chen, M.C. Chiu, An improved explainable artificial intelligence tool in healthcare for hospital recommendation. Healthcare Anal. **3**, 100147 (2023)
54. T. Chen, C. Ou, Y.C. Lin, A fuzzy polynomial fitting and mathematical programming approach for enhancing the accuracy and precision of productivity forecasting. Comput. Math. Organ. Theory **25**, 85–107 (2019)
55. Y.C. Wang, T. Chen, New XAI tools for selecting suitable 3D printing facilities in ubiquitous manufacturing. Compl. Intell. Syst. **9**, 6813–6829 (2023)
56. B. Ghai, Q.V. Liao, Y. Zhang, R. Bellamy, K. Mueller, Explainable active learning (xal): an empirical study of how local explanations impact annotator experience. arXiv preprint arXiv: 2001.09219 (2020)
57. T.C.T. Chen, in *Advances in Fuzzy Group Decision Making*. Deriving the Priorities of Criteria (2021), pp. 29–53.
58. S. Bassan, G. Katz, in *International Conference on Tools and Algorithms for the Construction and Analysis of Systems*. Towards Formal XAI: Formally Approximate Minimal Explanations of Neural Networks (2023), pp. 187–207
59. T.C.T. Chen, Y.C. Wang, M.C. Chiu, An efficient approximating alpha-cut operations approach for deriving fuzzy priorities in fuzzy multi-criterion decision-making. Appl. Soft Comput. **139**, 110238 (2023)
60. A.M. Antoniadi, Y. Du, Y. Guendouz, L. Wei, C. Mazo, B.A. Becker, C. Mooney, Current challenges and future opportunities for XAI in machine learning-based clinical decision support systems: a systematic review. Appl. Sci. **11**(11), 5088 (2021)
61. Y.C. Lin, T. Chen, A ubiquitous clinic recommendation system using the modified mixed-binary nonlinear programming-feedforward neural network approach. J. Theor. Appl. Electron. Commer. Res. **16**(7), 3282–3298 (2021)
62. T.C.T. Chen, C.W. Lin, Assessing cloud manufacturing applications using an optimally rectified FAHP approach. Compl. Intell. Syst. **8**(6), 5087–5099 (2022)
63. H.C. Wu, T. Chen, C.H. Huang, A piecewise linear FGM approach for efficient and accurate FAHP analysis: smart backpack design as an example. Mathematics **8**(8), 1319 (2020)
64. Y.C. Wang, T.C.T. Chen, A partial-consensus posterior-aggregation FAHP method—supplier selection problem as an example. Mathematics **7**(2), 179 (2019)

Chapter 3
XAmI Applications to Smart Homes

Abstract A smart home is an environment where users spend most of their time. However, unlike location-aware systems or telemedicine or telecare systems, smart homes can be controlled by the user, even from the outside. Therefore, assisting users in operating smart home appliances has become a key task. To accomplish this task, various sensors and actuators are installed in smart home appliances to detect user conditions and needs, accompanied by many artificial intelligence (AI) applications. This chapter first summarizes the applications of AI technologies in smart homes. Explainable ambient intelligence (XAmI) techniques can then be applied to extract useful behavioral patterns of users from these AI applications, thereby making such AI applications more autonomous and intelligent. Common XAmI techniques for this purpose include fuzzy inference rules, decision rules (or trees), random forests, and locally interpretable model-agnostic explanations (LIME).

Keywords Smart home · Explainable artificial intelligence · Locally interpretable model-agnostic explanations · Fuzzy inference rules

3.1 Artificial Intelligence (AI) Applications in Smart Homes

A smart home (or smart house) is a special environment in which the user spends most of their time, but which can be controlled from the outside. As an important application of ambient intelligence (AmI), artificial intelligence (AI) technologies have been widely used to support users' smart home life. The first AI technology is fuzzy logic. Zhang et al. [1] built a fuzzy expert system that considers sunlight, electrical quality, wind, and the power of uncontrollable and controllable loads to manage energy consumption in a smart home. The fuzzy inference system used in their study is the Mamdani fuzzy inference system (FIS) [2–3]. Similar systems have been widely installed in many smart home appliances, which can be controlled through the smart home console.

Example 3.1 A smart air conditioner automatically adjusts the fan speed after sensing room temperature and humidity. To this end, the following fuzzy inference rules are established:

Rule 1: If *room temperature* is "very high" And *humidity* is "high" Then *fan speed* is "fast."
Rule 2: If *room temperature* is "low" Or *humidity* is "low" Then *fan speed* is "slow."
Rule 3: If *humidity* is "very high" Then *fan speed* is "medium."

The membership functions of the linguistic terms in these rules are shown in Fig. 3.1. These rules form a Mamdani FIS [4–5].

Fig. 3.1 Membership functions of linguistic terms

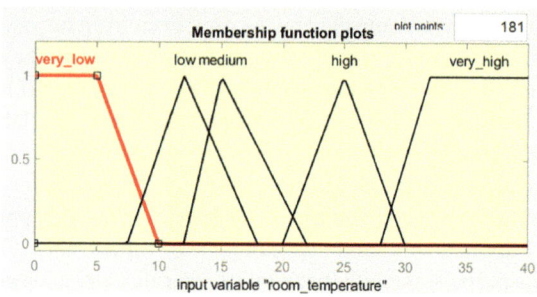

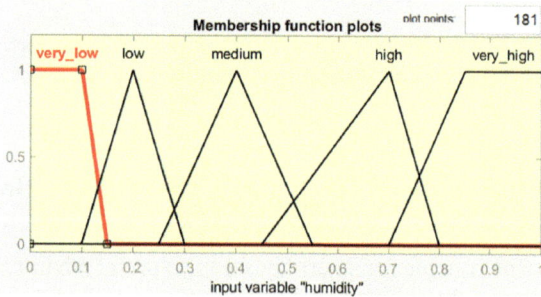

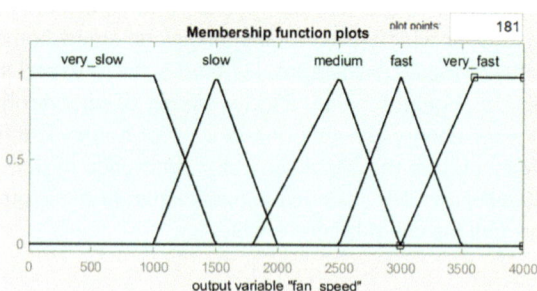

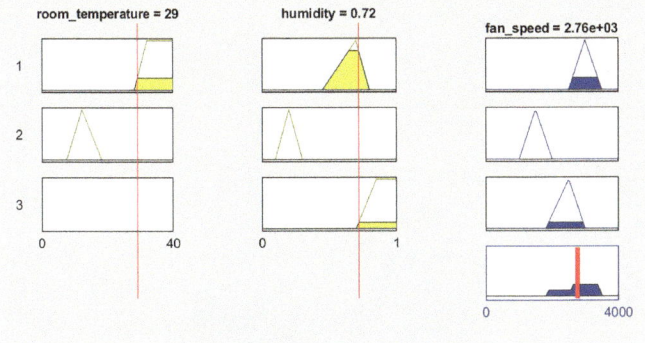

Fig. 3.2 Control result using the Mamdani FIS

According to the monitoring result of sensors in the smart home, the (average) room temperature is 29 °C and the (average) humidity is 72%. After applying the FIS, the fan speed is set to 2760 rpm, as illustrated in Fig. 3.2. The response surface is shown in Fig. 3.3.

Artificial neural networks (ANNs) [6–7] are another AI technology widely used in smart homes [8–10]. Badlani and Bhanot [11] constructed a recurrent neural network (RNN) to set the states of four smart home appliances (fans, air conditioners, light bulbs, and desk lamps) based on the sensed room temperature and humidity. The raw data contained records manually set by users to understand user behavior. RNNs are similar to feedforward neural networks (FNNs), except that each layer in RNN has a recurrent connection with a delay associated with it. Every smart home appliance has two states, high or low. The RNN had a total of eight outputs.

Example 3.2 The room temperature, humidity, and the manual setting of a smart air conditioner have been recorded. The raw data is summarized in Table 3.1. An RNN is built to fit the relationship between the manual setting (i.e., temperature) of the smart air conditioner and the other two variables. The MALAB code for implementing the RNN is shown in Fig. 3.4. The RNN has one hidden layer with ten nodes; input delay is 2 (see Fig. 3.5). The Levenberg–Marquardt (LM) algorithm [12] is applied to train the RNN. The first 75 records are used to train the RNN, while the remaining is left for evaluation. The forecasting results are compared with actual values in Fig. 3.6. The forecasting accuracy, in terms of root mean squared error (RMSE), is 1.38 °C:

$$\text{RMSE} = \sqrt{\sum_{t=1}^{T} (o_t - a_t)^2} \tag{3.1}$$

which is small and means that the RNN does approximate the user's behavior in setting the smart air conditioner. The performance of an AI application usually serves as a **global explanation** [13–14] of the AI application.

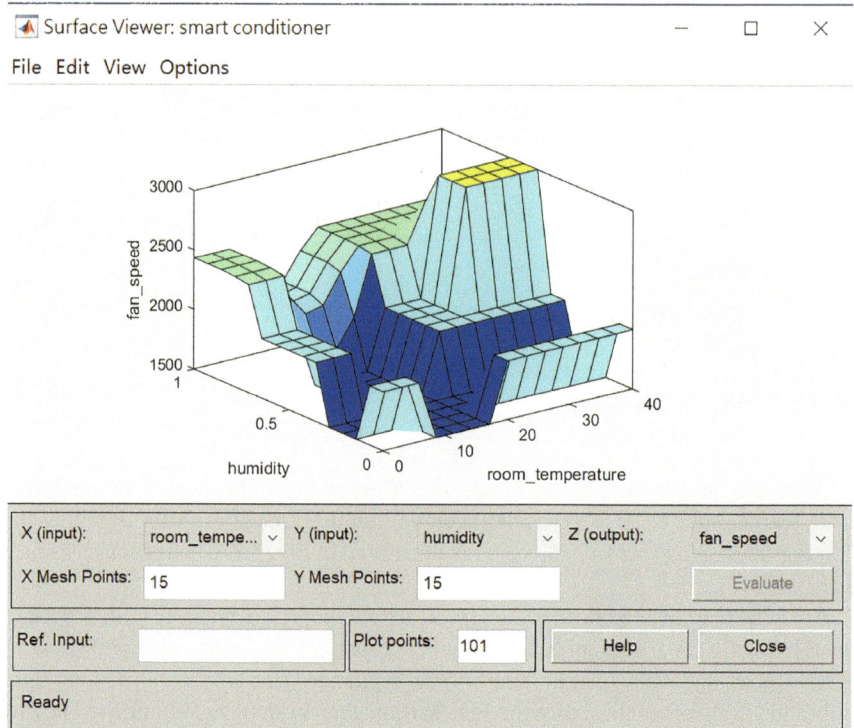

Fig. 3.3 Response surface of the Mamdani FIS

Table 3.1 Room temperature, humidity, and the manual setting of a smart air conditioner

Record no. (t)	Room temperature	Humidity (%)	Manual setting (a_t)
1	19	54	25
2	18	50	27
3	19	52	27
...			
100	29	55	26

When room temperature is 29 °C and humidity is 72%, the setting of the smart air conditioner predicted using the RNN is 28.14 °C (see Fig. 3.7).

Smart home appliances can be divided into two major categories: removable home appliances and non-removable home appliances. The former plays an important role in demand-side load management because they can be scheduled based on the real-time pricing (RTP) signal from the utility, while the latter is not as important in load management because these home appliances are fixed and unable to schedule based on RTP [15]. Hussain et al. [15] formulated a mathematical programming model to

```
X1=[19 0.54; 18 0.5; 19 0.52; ...; 30 0.61];
T1=[25; 27; 27; ...; 26];
X2=[30 0.65; 30 0.69; 29 0.73; ...; 29 0.55];
T2=[26; 24; 25; ...; 26];
X1=transpose(X1);
T1=transpose(T1);
X2=transpose(X2);
T2=transpose(T2);
% con2seq: Convert concurrent vectors to sequential vectors
X1=con2seq(X1);
T1=con2seq(T1);
X2=con2seq(X2);
T2=con2seq(T2);

net=layrecnet(1:2, 10);
[Xs1, Xi1, Ai1, Ts1]=preparets(net, X1, T1);
[Xs2, Xi2, Ai2, Ts2]=preparets(net, X2, T2);
net=train(net, Xs1, Ts1, Xi1, Ai1);
Y1=net(Xs1, Xi1, Ai1);
Y2=net(Xs2, Xi2, Ai2);
```

Fig. 3.4 MATLAB code for implementing the RNN

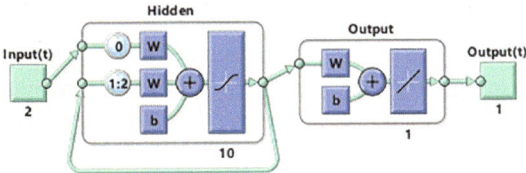

Fig. 3.5 Architecture of the RNN

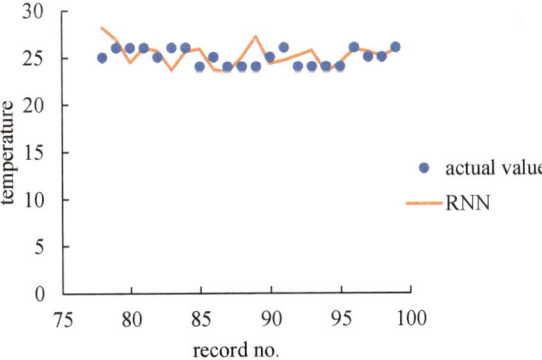

Fig. 3.6 Forecasting results

```
>> net([29;0.72],{},{})

ans =

    28.1408
```

Fig. 3.7 Prediction result using the RNN

minimize the total cost of energy consumption in smart homes. To solve this problem, they applied and compared two algorithms: the dragonfly algorithm and the genetic algorithm (GA) [16]. According to the experimental results, the dragonfly algorithm was more capable of smoothing out hourly load fluctuations.

Preventing falls among the elderly is an important task for smart homes. Correct detection can reduce the deaths and injuries of the elderly, while incorrect detection will lead to incorrect dispatch and waste of rescue resources. To this end, Yu et al. [17] established a fall detection system based on posture recognition, in which a directed acyclic graph support vector machine (SVM) [18–19] was applied for posture classification. Experimental results showed that the fall detection system based on gesture recognition achieved a high fall detection rate and an extremely low false detection rate.

It is not easy to choose a suitable smart home application for fall detection. To address this issue, Lin et al. [20] proposed a fuzzy collaborative intelligence approach, in which alpha-cut operations were applied to derive the fuzzy weights of criteria for each surveillance person. Then, fuzzy intersection was applied to aggregate the fuzzy weights derived by all surveillance persons. Subsequently, the fuzzy technique for order preference by similarity to the ideal solution (TOPSIS) [21–22] was applied to assess the suitability of a smart home application for fall detection. The fuzzy collaborative intelligence approach was a posterior-aggregation method that guaranteed a consensus exists among surveillance persons.

Wang et al. [23] classified existing fall detection systems in smart homes into four categories: systems based on ambient devices, systems based on vision, systems based on wearable devices, and systems based on smartphones. Measures to evaluate the performance of fall detection systems include accuracy, false alarm rate, and efficiency [23]. In contrast, Mubashir et al. [24] listed five criteria for selecting a suitable smart home application for fall detection: low cost, unobtrusive, accurate, easy to set up, and robust.

De Lima et al. [25] attached various sensors (or sensor combinations), including three-axis accelerometers, force and bending sensors, and gyroscopes, to the chests, insoles, and lower backs of older adults in smart homes to find the best smart sensor application for fall detection. In contrast, Li et al. [26] installed two sensors on the chests and right thighs of smart home residents. Each sensor consisted of a three-axis accelerometer and a three-axis gyroscope. An algorithm for detecting a resident's fall based on readings from two sensors was proposed. If the resident carries a smartphone, the surveillance person can also use the smartphone for fall detection by analyzing the accelerometer and gyroscope readings on the smartphone.

However, this was a challenging task because the resident's gesture and movement were diverse and constantly changing. To solve this problem, the joint use of smart watches and smartphones was adopted [27–28], where the smart watch sensed the resident's gesture and movement, while the smartphone inferred and communicated with the surveillance person, which was more effective than using smartphones alone [29].

Smart homes are usually equipped with smart surveillance systems. Taking advantage of this, Senouci et al. [30] designed a fall detection system based on smart cameras. Two classification methods, SVM and AdaBoost, were applied to analyze the recorded images. Experimental results show that for fall detection, SVM achieved higher classification accuracy, while AdaBoost was more efficient. From the viewpoint of Wang et al. [23], the wireless signal in a smart home was affected by resident motions in the smart home, which could be utilized to detect a fall.

According to Ojetola et al. [31], the difficulties in applying fall detection technologies in smart homes include setting thresholds to distinguish falls from non-falls, generalizing the algorithm to other subject groups, validation of the method (or system), and real-time detection. In addition, the disruption caused by installing additional hardware may become an obstacle to widespread deployment of fall detection systems in smart homes. Optimizing smart home applications for fall detection is a more difficult task. Furthermore, the quality of the sensory data is undoubtedly critical to the effectiveness of the subsequent analysis and decision-making processes [32–33].

Chen [34] proposed the fuzzy geometric mean (FGM)-alpha-cut operations (ACO)-fuzzy weighted average (FWA) method to evaluate the sustainability of a smart home application for fall detection, in which surveillance persons' judgments were aggregated using FGM before deriving the fuzzy weights of criteria using ACO.

The data collected by sensors in smart homes is obviously big data, which makes it difficult to extract useful patterns of resident behavior [35–36]. Time series data can be replaced by its statistics (such as mean and standard deviation) to reduce volume. The number of inputs to an AI application in smart homes can be reduced by eliminating dependencies between them to form fewer new variables.

There are at least three methods in the literature to consider dependencies between the inputs to an AI application in smart homes: the analytical network process (ANP) approach [37], the principal component analysis (PCA) approach [38], and the quality function deployment (QFD) approach [39]. ANP is an extension of analytic hierarchy process (AHP). In ANP, a supermatrix of pairwise comparisons is constructed (see Fig. 3.8). An input may have different importance levels for different smart home applications. Therefore, dependencies between inputs are subjective and may not be easily quantified:

$$\tilde{\chi}_j = f_{\text{ANP}}(\{\tilde{x}_i\}) \tag{3.2}$$

Supermatrix		Applications			Inputs		
		A_1	A_2	A_3	x_1	x_2	x_3
Applications	P_1	Relative performance of application k to application l			Performance of application k with regard to input j		
	P_2						
	P_3						
Inputs	x_1	Importance of input i to application l			Relative importance of input i to input j		
	x_2						
	x_3						

Fig. 3.8 Pairwise comparison supermatrix

Furthermore, it becomes pointless to derive a new set of variables for all applications. FGM can be used to process a pairwise comparison supermatrix [40]. In this way, the values of new variables can be derived and applications simultaneously evaluated.

In PCA, PCA extracts independent inputs through a linear combination of the original inputs, and then the value of the new input is equal to the same linear combination of the original values:

$$\tilde{\chi}_j = \sum_{i=1}^{n} \beta_i \tilde{x}_i \tag{3.3}$$

$$r_{\tilde{\chi}_j, \tilde{\chi}_k} = 0 \quad \forall j \neq k \tag{3.4}$$

In QFD, new independent variables are defined by combining the original inputs using prespecified rules [41–42] (see Fig. 3.9). These rules, whether linear or nonlinear, can be quantified. Dependencies between the original inputs are also considered. Then, pairwise comparisons are performed on the new variables. However, the first way is purely subjective, and in other respects, the overall performance of AI applications in smart homes does not directly map to the original inputs, which is not in line with the trend of XAmI.

Autoencoders (AEs) [43] can also be used to solve the problem of analyzing big data collected by smart home sensors. An AE is a symmetrical neural network whose output goal is to reproduce input samples to learn representations of latent features. The basic architecture of the autoencoder is shown in Fig. 3.10. It includes input layer, hidden layer, and output layer. The encoder part converts the original inputs $\{x_{jp}\}$ into new (latent) variables $\{h_{jq}\}$:

$$\text{Encoder}: \mathbf{h_j} = \sigma(\mathbf{w_1 x_j} + \mathbf{b_x}); \; j = 1 \sim n \tag{3.5}$$

	Original input 1	Original input 2	Original input 3
New input 1	⊙	⊙	○
New input 2	△	⊙	○
New input 3	○	○	⊙

⊙: Strong
○: Medium
△: Weak

Fig. 3.9 Establishing new criteria from the original criteria using QFD

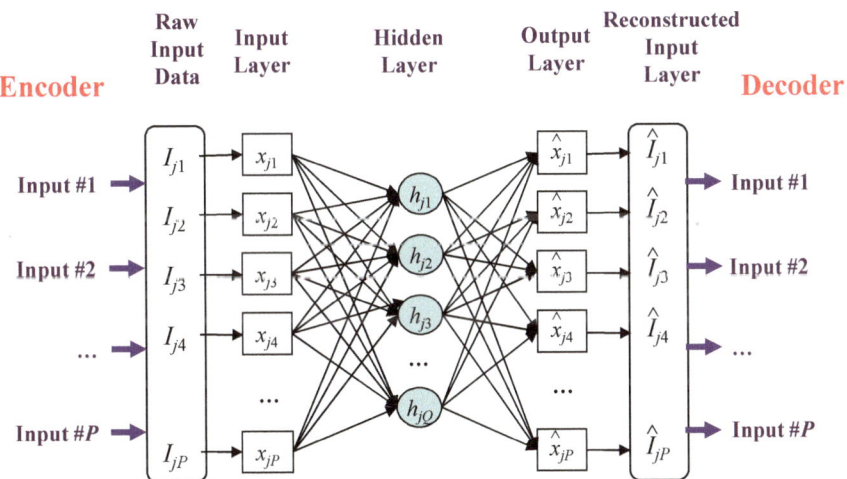

Fig. 3.10 Basic architecture of an AE

In contrast, the output layer is a decoder that reconstructs latent features to approximate the values of inputs:

$$\text{Decoder} : \hat{\mathbf{x}}_{\mathbf{j}} = \sigma'(\mathbf{w}_2 \mathbf{h}_{\mathbf{j}} + \mathbf{b}_{\mathbf{h}}); \ j = 1 \sim n \tag{3.6}$$

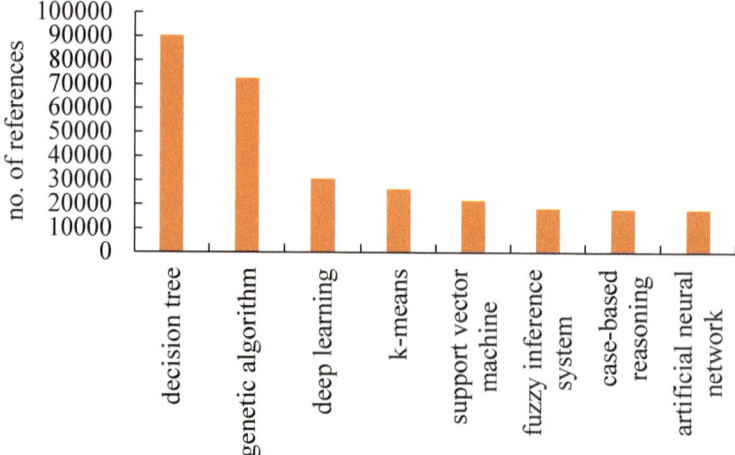

Fig. 3.11 Number of references about AI technology applications in smart homes from 2010 to 2023 (Data source Google Scholar)

However, some question that this variable substitution may make it difficult to assess the impact of various inputs on the output. Nonetheless, existing XAmI techniques are still theoretically suitable for handling this situation.

Figure 3.11 provides statistics on the popularity of AI technology applications in smart homes. AI technologies most widely used in smart homes include decision trees (DTs), GAs, and deep learning [44–45].

3.2   XAmI Technique for Explaining Fuzzy Logic Applications in Smart Homes

Although users do not know the values set by a smart home appliance for the linguistic terms, they are certain of these values. Therefore, fuzzy inference rules, like decision rules, do not require interpretation. However, this only applies to fuzzy inference rules based on ordinary fuzzy sets. Fuzzy inference rules based on advanced fuzzy sets, such as type-II fuzzy sets [46–47], Fermatean fuzzy sets [48–49], intuitionistic fuzzy sets [50–51], fuzzy rough sets [52–53], and hesitant fuzzy sets [54–56], still require explanations. An intuitive approach is to explain such fuzzy inference rules with simpler fuzzy inference rules with ordinary fuzzy sets [57–58].

3.3 XAmI Technique for Explaining ANN Applications in Smart Homes

3.3.1 Interpretable Model-Agnostic Explanation (LIME)

When explaining ANN applications in smart homes, one can follow the idea of locally interpretable model-agnostic explanation (LIME) [59], which is to approximate the ANN application (black-box model) with a locally interpretable model to explain each individual prediction. To this end, synthetic data needs to be generated from the original data to avoid the impact of extreme or exceptional cases and missing data [60–61]. However, such synthetic data has no actual values.

Example 3.3 For Example 3.2, the synthetic data is generated from the original data by randomizing the room temperature (x_{s1}) and humidity (x_{s2}) values:

(Randomization Mechanism for RNNs)

$$x_{s1} = x_{s-1,1} + RN_{r1} \cdot \min_r(x_{r1} - x_{r-1,1})$$
$$+ (1 - RN_{r1}) \cdot \max_r(x_{r1} - x_{r-1,1}) \tag{3.7}$$

$$x_{s2} = x_{s-1,2} + RN_{r2} \cdot \min_r(x_{r2} - x_{r-1,2})$$
$$+ (1 - RN_{r2}) \cdot \max_r(x_{r2} - x_{r-1,2}) \tag{3.8}$$

where x_{r1} and x_{r1} denote the room temperature and humidity values in the raw data. RN_{r1} and RN_{r2} are random numbers in [0, 1]. It is worth noting that RNNs use a different randomization mechanism than feedforward neural networks (FNNs) because the data is time series correlated [62–63]:

(Randomization Mechanism for FNNs)

$$x_{s1} = RN_{r1} \cdot \min_r x_{r1} + (1 - RN_{r1}) \cdot \max_r x_{r1} \tag{3.9}$$

$$x_{s2} = RN_{r2} \cdot \min_r x_{r2} + (1 - RN_{r2}) \cdot \max_r x_{r2} \tag{3.10}$$

The synthetic data contains 200 records, as shown in Table 3.2. For each record, the trained RNN is used to predict the manual setting (i.e., temperature) of the smart air conditioner. The required MATLAB code is shown in Fig. 3.12. The forecasting results are indicated with o_s's, $s = 1 \sim 200$.

Table 3.2 Synthetic data

Record no	Room temperature	Humidity (%)	o_s
1	25	54	–
2	25	50	–
3	23	52	27
...			
200	17	23	25

```
X3=[25 0.54; 25 0.50; 23 0.52; ...; 17 0.23];
X3=transpose(X3);
X3=con2seq(X3);
[Xs3, Xi3, Ai3, Ts3]=preparets(net, X3, {});
Y3=net(Xs3, Xi3, Ai3);
```

Fig. 3.12 MATLAB code for applying the trained RNN to synthetic data

3.3.2 LIME + Decision Trees (DTs)

The RNN can then be fitted using simpler machine learning models such as decision trees (DTs) [64–65], random forests (RFs) [66–67], and fuzzy inference rules [68–69] (see Fig. 3.13).

Example 3.4 A DT is constructed to approximate the RNN for smart air conditioner control in Example 3.2 based on the synthetic data generated in Example 3.3. The required MATLAB code is shown in Fig. 3.14. The constructed DT is illustrated in Fig. 3.15, with decision rules summarized in Fig. 3.16. There are 40 rules in this

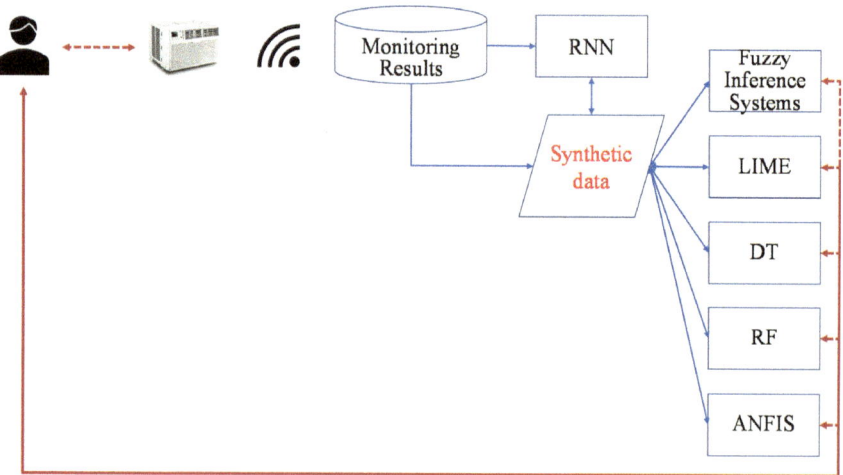

Fig. 3.13 Various ways to fit the RNN

```
% Approximate the RNN with a DT
X3=[25 0.54; 25 0.50; 23 0.52; ...; 17 0.23];
T3=[28; 27; 25; ...; 25];
DT1=fitrtree(X3(3:200,:), T3);
view(DT1, 'Mode', 'text');
view(DT1, 'Mode', 'graph');
osh=predict(DT1, X3(3:200,:));
mean((osh-T3).^2)^0.5
```

Fig. 3.14 MATLAB code for approximating the RNN with a DT

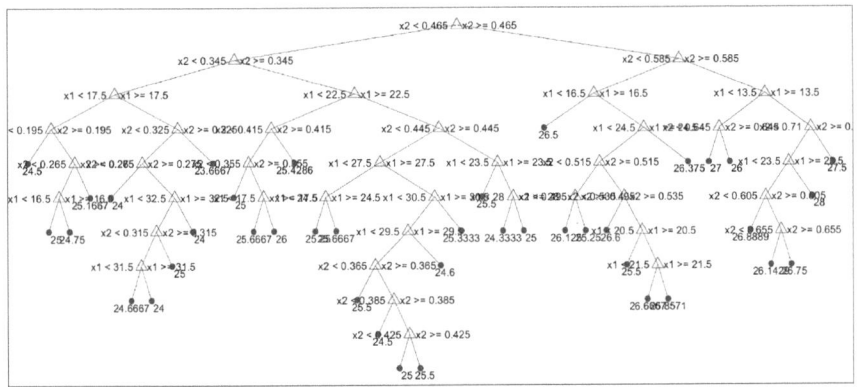

Fig. 3.15 DT constructed for approximating the RNN

case. For each sensing result, only one decision rule is applicable. For example, when room temperature is 29 °C and humidity is 72%, the decision rule applicable is:

$$\text{If } x_1 \geq 13.5 \text{ and } x_2 \geq 0.71 \text{ Then } \hat{o}_s = 27.5.$$

while $o_j = 28.1$ (°C), which is quite close. After removing technical terms.

"If room temperature is higher than or equal to 13.5 °C, and humidity is above or equal to 71%, then the setting of smart air conditioner is 27.5 °C." This is a **local explanation**.

1	if x2<0.465 then node 2 elseif x2>=0.465 then node 3 else 25.5707
2	if x2<0.345 then node 4 elseif x2>=0.345 then node 5 else 25.0175
3	if x2<0.585 then node 6 elseif x2>=0.585 then node 7 else 26.3214
4	if x1<17.5 then node 8 elseif x1>=17.5 then node 9 else 24.6809
5	if x1<22.5 then node 10 elseif x1>=22.5 then node 11 else 25.2537
6	if x1<16.5 then node 12 elseif x1>=16.5 then node 13 else 26.0851
...	
77	if x2<0.425 then node 78 elseif x2>=0.425 then node 79 else 25.1
78	fit = 25
79	fit = 25.5

Fig. 3.16 Decision rules of the DT

The explanation performance can be evaluated in terms of the RMSE of approximating o_s with $\hat{o}_s$:

$$\text{RMSE} = \sqrt{\sum_{s=1}^{S} (o_s - \hat{o}_s)^2} \tag{3.11}$$

In Example 3.4, RMSE is 1.68 °C. The explanation performance can be further enhanced using a RF. Other performance measures for this purpose include mean absolute error (MAE), mean absolute percentage error (MAPE), and coefficient of determination (R^2):

$$\text{MAE} = \frac{1}{S} \sum_{s=1}^{S} |o_s - \hat{o}_s| \tag{3.12}$$

$$\text{MAPE} = \frac{1}{S} \sum_{s=1}^{S} \frac{|o_s - \hat{o}_s|}{o_s} \cdot 100\% \tag{3.13}$$

$$R^2 = 1 - \frac{\sum_{s=1}^{S} (o_s - \hat{o}_s)^2}{\sum_{s=1}^{S} (o_s - \overline{o}_s)^2} \tag{3.14}$$

3.3.3   LIME + Random Forests (RFs)

However, people's feelings and preferences are constantly changing [70], which is also reflected in the requirements and controls of smart home appliances. Therefore, a single DT may not be accurate enough to approximate ANN applications in smart homes. To solve this problem, a RF composed of several DTs can be constructed. Each decision tree considers a random subset of attributes (i.e., feature bagging) and is trained with examples randomly selected from the data with replacement (i.e., bootstrapping) [71–72]. In each DT, there is a decision rule that applies to a certain control action. The outcomes of the decision rules in all DTs applicable to the control action are averaged to generate a representative forecast.

Example 3.5 (LIME Application with RF) A RF composed of 10 DTs is constructed instead to approximate the RNN for smart air conditioner control in Example 3.2 based on the synthetic data generated in Example 3.3. The required MATLAB code is shown in Fig. 3.17. The constructed RF is illustrated in Fig. 3.18, with decision rules summarized in Fig. 3.19. RMSE = 1.28 °C, much better than that achieved when a single DT is used to fit the RNN.

```
% Approximate the RNN with a RF
X3=[25 0.54; 25 0.50; 23 0.52; ...; 17 0.23];
T3=[28; 27; 25; ...; 25];
RF1=TreeBagger(10, X3(3:200,:), transpose(T3), Method="regression", OOBPrediction="on");
osh=predict(RF1, X3(3:200,:));
mean((osh-T3).^2)^0.5

% Show the first DT
view(RF1.Trees{1},'Mode','graph');
view(RF1.Trees{1},'Mode','text');
```

Fig. 3.17 MATLAB code for approximating the RNN with a RF

3.3.4 LIME + Fuzzy Inference Rules

As mentioned before, the linguistic terms in fuzzy inference rules are interpretable and require no further explanation [73–74]. Therefore, fuzzy inference rules, like decision rules, can be applied to interpret black-box models, such as artificial neural networks, without the need for explanation. An adaptive network-based fuzzy inference system (ANFIS), as a hybrid of ANNs and FISs, is actually an automatic tool for extracting fuzzy inference rules from the collected data or black-box models [75–76]. Therefore, the following example applies ANFIS to extract fuzzy inference rules from the ANN for controlling a smart home appliance.

Example 3.6 (LIME Application with Fuzzy Inference Rules) An ANFIS is constructed to extract fuzzy inference rules from the RNN for smart air conditioner control in Example 3.2. The ranges of all variables (i.e., room temperature, humidity, and manual setting) are fuzzily divided into five equal intervals, represented by corresponding linguistic terms, as shown in Example 3.1. Then, all possible combinations of variable values form fuzzy inference rules. The support and confidence of each fuzzy inference rule are evaluated [77–78]. Only fuzzy inference rules with sufficiently high support and confidence remain. The required MATLAB code is shown in Fig. 3.20. The membership functions of the fuzzy numbers of inputs are shown in Fig. 3.21. RMSE = 1.14 °C. When room temperature is 29 °C and humidity is 72%, the estimated setting is 27.9 °C (see Fig. 3.22), while $o_j = 28.1$ (°C), which is quite close. The response surface is shown in Fig. 3.23, which is more complex than that in Fig. 3.3, showing a more precise control.

However, training an ANFIS will be a time-consuming task if each input (i.e., monitored condition) is divided into many fuzzy intervals [79–83]. In addition, there are many ways to divide an input, which makes the optimization of the ANFIS another difficult task. Furthermore, the combinations of all inputs contribute to a lot of rules, few of which are supported by the monitoring results.

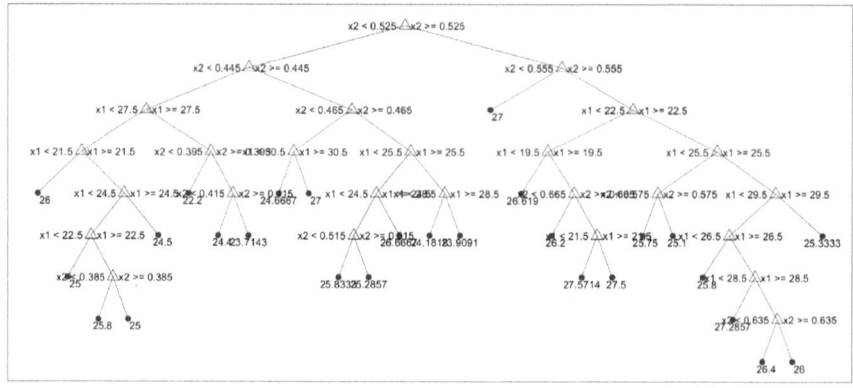

(2nd DT)

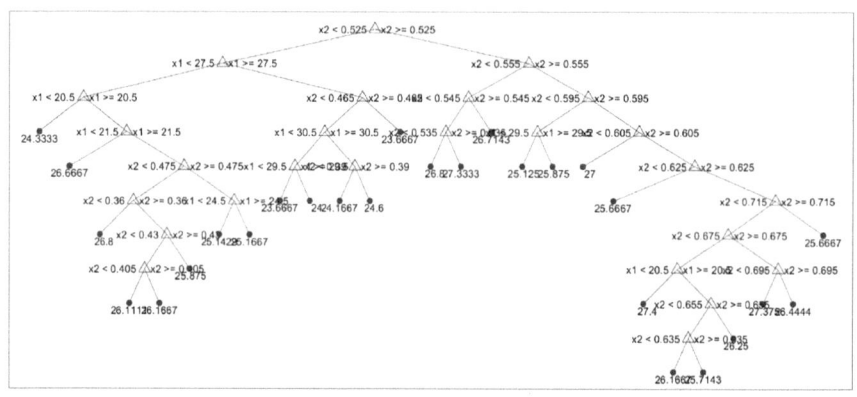

...

(10th DT)

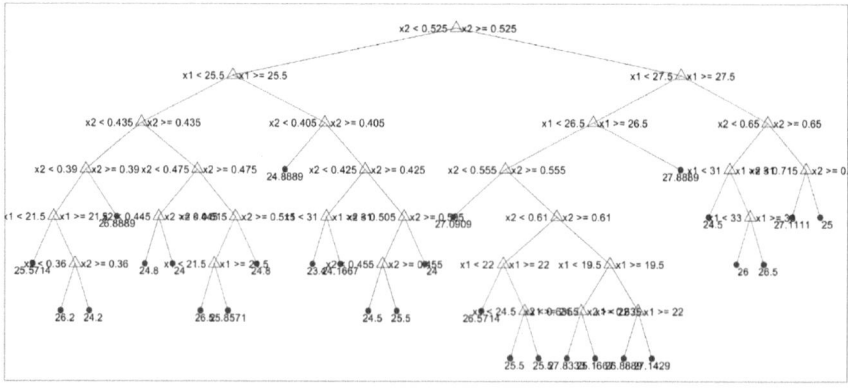

Fig. 3.18   RF constructed for approximating the RNN

(1st DT)
1 if x2<0.525 then node 2 elseif x2>=0.525 then node 3 else 25.6061
2 if x2<0.445 then node 4 elseif x2>=0.445 then node 5 else 24.8713
3 if x2<0.555 then node 6 elseif x2>=0.555 then node 7 else 26.3711
4 if x1<27.5 then node 8 elseif x1>=27.5 then node 9 else 24.6531
5 if x2<0.465 then node 10 elseif x2>=0.465 then node 11 else 25.0769
6 fit = 27
...
51 if x2<0.635 then node 52 elseif x2>=0.635 then node 53 else 26.2
52 fit = 26.4
53 fit = 26

(2nd DT)
1 if x2<0.525 then node 2 elseif x2>=0.525 then node 3 else 25.7525
2 if x1<27.5 then node 4 elseif x1>=27.5 then node 5 else 25.0825
3 if x2<0.555 then node 6 elseif x2>=0.555 then node 7 else 26.396
4 if x1<20.5 then node 8 elseif x1>=20.5 then node 9 else 25.7458
5 if x2<0.465 then node 10 elseif x2>=0.465 then node 11 else 24.0526
6 if x2<0.545 then node 12 elseif x2>=0.545 then node 13 else 26.9444
...
51 fit = 26.25
52 fit = 26.1667
53 fit = 25.7143

...

(10th DT)
1 if x2<0.525 then node 2 elseif x2>=0.525 then node 3 else 25.7677
2 if x1<25.5 then node 4 elseif x1>=25.5 then node 5 else 25.0833
3 if x1<27.5 then node 6 elseif x1>=27.5 then node 7 else 26.4118
4 if x2<0.435 then node 8 elseif x2>=0.435 then node 9 else 25.5455
5 if x2<0.405 then node 10 elseif x2>=0.405 then node 11 else 24.4634
6 if x1<26.5 then node 12 elseif x1>=26.5 then node 13 else 26.7313
...
55 fit = 25.1667
56 fit = 26.8889
57 fit = 27.1429

Fig. 3.19 Decision rules of the RF

```
% Approximate the RNN with an ANFIS
X3=[25 0.54; 25 0.50; 23 0.52; ... ; 17 0.23];
T3=[28; 27; 25; ... ; 25];
opt=genfisOptions('GridPartition');
opt.NumMembershipFunctions=[5 5];
opt.InputMembershipFunctionType=["trimf" "trimf"];
fis1=genfis(X3(3:200,:), T3, opt);
fis1=anfis([X3(3:200,:) T3], fis1);

% Show the fuzzy numbers
[x,mf]=plotmf(fis1, 'input', 1);
subplot(2, 1, 1);
plot(x, mf);
xlabel('room temperature (triangular)');
ylabel('membership');
[x,mf]=plotmf(fis1, 'input', 2);
subplot(2, 1, 2);
plot(x, mf);
xlabel('humidity (triangular)');
ylabel('membership');
```

Fig. 3.20   MATLAB code for approximating the RNN with an ANFIS

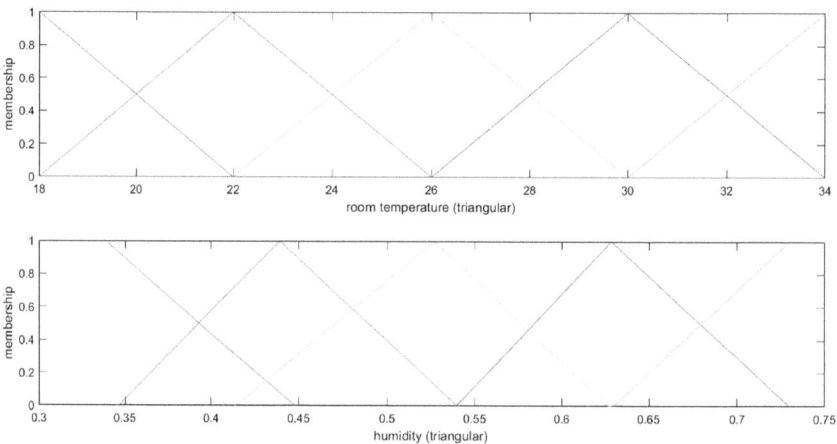

Fig. 3.21   Membership functions of the fuzzy numbers of inputs

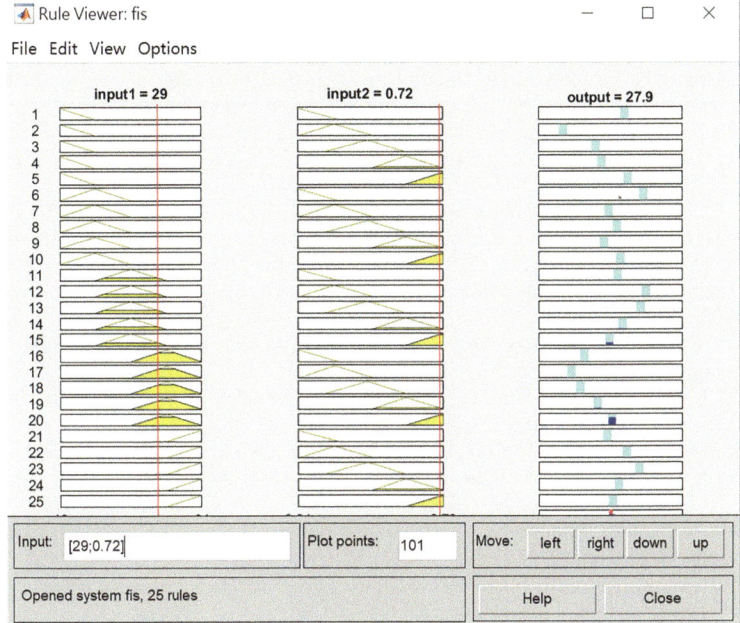

Fig. 3.22 Estimation result

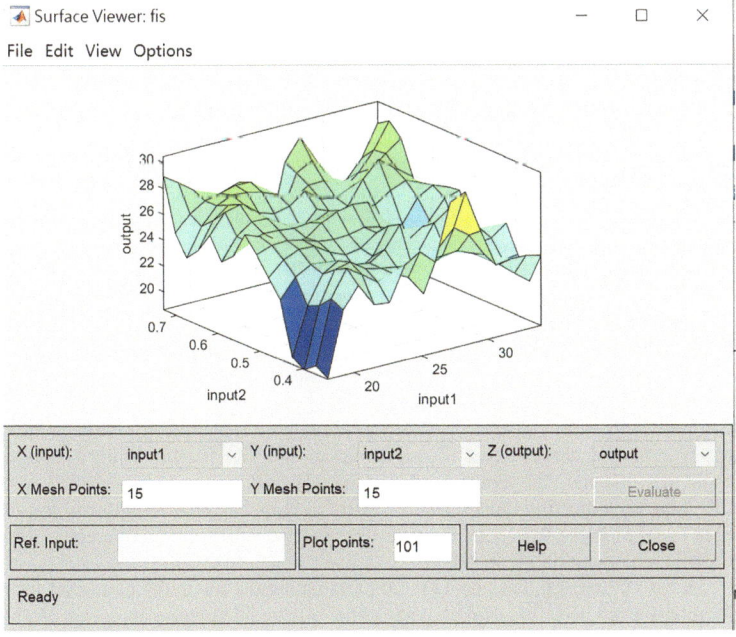

Fig. 3.23 Response surface

References

1. R. Zhang, V.E. Sathishkumar, R. Dinesh Jackson Samuel, Fuzzy efficient energy smart home management system for renewable energy resources. Sustainability **12**(8), 3115 (2020)
2. E. Pourjavad, R.V. Mayorga, A comparative study and measuring performance of manufacturing systems with Mamdani fuzzy inference system. J. Intell. Manuf. **30**(3), 1085–1097 (2019)
3. T.C.T. Chen, in *Sustainable Smart Healthcare: Lessons Learned from the COVID-19 Pandemic.* Enhancing the Sustainability of Smart Healthcare Applications with XAI (2023), pp. 93–110
4. K. Iqbal, M.A. Khan, S. Abbas, Z. Hasan, A. Fatima, Intelligent transportation system (ITS) for smart-cities using Mamdani fuzzy inference system. Int. J. Adv. Comput. Sci. Appl. **9**(2), 94–105 (2018)
5. T.C.T. Chen, in *Advances in Fuzzy Group Decision Making.* Introduction to Fuzzy Group Decision Making (2022), pp. 1–7
6. T.C.T. Chen, Y.C. Lin, Fuzzified deep neural network ensemble approach for estimating cycle time range. Appl. Soft Comput. **130**, 109697 (2022)
7. H.C. Wu, T.C.T. Chen, M.C. Chiu, Constructing a precise fuzzy feedforward neural network using an independent fuzzification approach. Axioms **10**(4), 282 (2021)
8. T.C.T. Chen, in *Sustainable Smart Healthcare: Lessons Learned from the COVID-19 Pandemic.* Smart Technology Applications in Healthcare Before, During, and After the COVID-19 Pandemic (2023), pp. 19–37
9. A. Hussein, M. Adda, M. Atieh, W. Fahs, Smart home design for disabled people based on neural networks. Proc. Comput. Sci. **37**, 117–126 (2014)
10. T.C.T. Chen, Y.C. Lin, Y.C. Wang, A heterogeneous fuzzy collaborative intelligence approach: air quality monitor selection study. Appl. Soft Comput. **149**, 111000 (2023)
11. A. Badlani, S. Bhanot, Smart home system design based on artificial neural networks. Proc. World Congr. Eng. Comput. Sci. **1**, 146–164 (2011)
12. S. Sapna, A. Tamilarasi, M.P. Kumar, Backpropagation learning algorithm based on Levenberg Marquardt Algorithm. Comput. Sci. Inf. Technol. **2**, 393–398 (2012)
13. T.C.T. Chen, C.W. Lin, Y.C. Lin, A fuzzy collaborative forecasting approach based on XAI applications for cycle time range estimation. Appl. Soft Comput. **151**, 111122 (2024)
14. Y.C. Wang, T.C.T. Chen, M.C. Chiu, A systematic approach to enhance the explainability of artificial intelligence in healthcare with application to diagnosis of diabetes. Healthcare Anal. **3**, 100183 (2023)
15. I. Hussain, M. Ullah, I. Ullah, A. Bibi, M. Naeem, M. Singh, D. Singh, Optimizing energy consumption in the home energy management system via a bio-inspired dragonfly algorithm and the genetic algorithm. Electronics **9**(3), 406 (2020)
16. T.C.T. Chen, Y.C. Wang, in *Artificial Intelligence and Lean Manufacturing.* AI Applications to Shop Floor Management in Lean Manufacturing (2022), pp. 75–90
17. M. Yu, A. Rhuma, S.M. Naqvi, L. Wang, J. Chambers, A posture recognition-based fall detection system for monitoring an elderly person in a smart home environment. IEEE Trans. Inf. Technol. Biomed. **16**(6), 1274–1286 (2012)
18. Y. Geng, J. Chen, R. Fu, G. Bao, K. Pahlavan, Enlighten wearable physiological monitoring systems: on-body rf characteristics based human motion classification using a support vector machine. IEEE Trans. Mob. Comput. **15**(3), 656–671 (2015)
19. T.C.T. Chen, in *Production Planning and Control in Semiconductor Manufacturing: Big Data Analytics and Industry 4.0 Applications.* Defect Pattern Analysis, Yield Learning Modeling, and Yield Prediction (2023), pp. 63–76
20. Y.C. Lin, Y.C. Wang, T.C.T. Chen, H.F. Lin, Evaluating the suitability of a smart technology application for fall detection using a fuzzy collaborative intelligence approach. Mathematics **7**(11), 1097 (2019)
21. Y. Çelikbilek, F. Tüysüz, An in-depth review of theory of the TOPSIS method: an experimental analysis. J. Manage. Anal. **7**(2), 281–300 (2020)

22. T. Chen, Y.C. Wang, P.H. Jiang, A selectively calibrated derivation technique and generalized fuzzy TOPSIS for semiconductor supply chain localization assessment. Decis. Anal. J. **8**, 100275 (2023)
23. Y. Wang, K. Wu, L.M. Ni, Wifall: device-free fall detection by wireless networks. IEEE Trans. Mob. Comput. **16**(2), 581–594 (2016)
24. M. Mubashir, L. Shao, L. Seed, A survey on fall detection: principles and approaches. Neurocomputing **100**, 144–152 (2013)
25. A.L.S. De Lima, L.J. Evers, T. Hahn, L. Bataille, J.L. Hamilton, M.A. Little, Y. Okuma, B.R. Bloem, M.J. Faber, Freezing of gait and fall detection in Parkinson's disease using wearable sensors: a systematic review. J. Neurol. **264**, 1642–1654 (2017)
26. Q. Li, J.A. Stankovic, M.A. Hanson, A.T. Barth, J. Lach, G. Zhou, in *2009 Sixth International Workshop on Wearable and Implantable Body Sensor Networks*. Accurate, Fast Fall Detection Using Gyroscopes and Accelerometer-Derived Posture Information (2009), pp. 138–143
27. T.C.T. Chen, in *Sustainable Smart Healthcare: Lessons Learned from the COVID-19 Pandemic*. Smart Healthcare (2023), pp. 1–18
28. E. Casilari, M.A. Oviedo-Jiménez, Automatic fall detection system based on the combined use of a smartphone and a smartwatch. PLoS ONE **10**(11), e0140929 (2015)
29. T.C.T. Chen, in *Sustainable Smart Healthcare: Lessons Learned from the COVID-19 Pandemic*. Sustainable Smart Healthcare Applications: Lessons Learned from the COVID-19 Pandemic (2023), pp. 65–92
30. B. Senouci, I. Charfi, B. Heyrman, J. Dubois, J. Miteran, Fast prototyping of a SoC-based smart-camera: a real-time fall detection case study. J. Real Time Image Process **12**, 649–662 (2016)
31. O. Ojetola, E.I. Gaura, J. Brusey, in *Proceedings of the 2011 Seventh International Conference on Intelligent Environments*. Fall Detection with Wearable Sensors—Safe (Smart Fall Detection) (2011), pp. 318–321.
32. T.C.T. Chen, M.C. Chiu, Evaluating the sustainability of smart technology applications in healthcare after the COVID-19 pandemic: a hybridising subjective and objective fuzzy group decision-making approach with explainable artificial intelligence. Digital Health **8**, 20552076221136380 (2022)
33. A. Leonardi, H. Ziekow, M. Strohbach, P. Kikiras, Dealing with data quality in smart home environments—lessons learned from a smart grid pilot. J. Sens. Actuator Netw. **5**(1), 5 (2016)
34. T.C.T. Chen, Evaluating the sustainability of a smart technology application to mobile health care: the FGM–ACO–FWA approach. Compl. Intell. Syst. **6**(1), 109–121 (2020)
35. A.R. Al-Ali, I.A. Zualkernan, M. Rashid, R. Gupta, M. AliKarar, A smart home energy management system using IoT and big data analytics approach. IEEE Trans. Consum. Electron. **63**(4), 426–434 (2017)
36. T.C.T. Chen, Big data analytics for semiconductor manufacturing. in *Production Planning and Control in Semiconductor Manufacturing: Big Data Analytics and Industry 4.0 Applications* (2022), pp. 1–19
37. P. Aragonés-Beltrán, F. Chaparro-González, J.P. Pastor-Ferrando, F. Rodríguez-Pozo, An ANP-based approach for the selection of photovoltaic solar power plant investment projects. Renew. Sustain. Energy Rev. **14**(1), 249–264 (2010)
38. R.A. Johnson, D.W. Wichern, *Applied Multivariate Statistical Analysis* (Prentice-Hall, 2007)
39. Y.C. Wang, T.C.T. Chen, Analyzing the impact of COVID-19 vaccination requirements on travelers' selection of hotels using a fuzzy multi-criteria decision-making approach. Healthcare Anal. **2**, 100064 (2022)
40. L. Mikhailov, M.G. Singh, Fuzzy analytic network process and its application to the development of decision support systems. IEEE Trans. Syst. Man Cybern. Part C **33**(1), 33–41 (2003)
41. T.C.T. Chen, T.C. Chang, Y.C. Wang, Improving people's health by burning low-pollution coal to improve air quality for thermal power generation. Digital Health **9**, 20552076231185280 (2023)

42. D. Buakum, C. Daesa, R. Sinthavalai, K. Noppasri, Designing temperature-controlled medicine bag using an integrated AHP-QFD methodology. Int. J. Inter. Design Manuf. 1–12 (2023)
43. J., Zhai, S., Zhang, J., Chen, & Q. He, in *2018 IEEE International Conference on Systems, Man, and Cybernetics*. Autoencoder and its Various Variants (2018), pp. 415–419
44. T.C.T. Chen, C.W. Lin, An FGM decomposition-based fuzzy MCDM method for selecting smart technology applications to support mobile health care during and after the COVID-19 pandemic. Appl. Soft Comput. **121**, 108758 (2022)
45. Y.C. Wang, T.C.T. Chen, H.C. Wu, A novel auto-weighting deep-learning fuzzy collaborative intelligence approach. Decis. Anal. J. **6**, 100186 (2023)
46. J. Qin, X. Liu, W. Pedrycz, An extended VIKOR method based on prospect theory for multiple attribute decision making under interval type-2 fuzzy environment. Knowl. Based Syst. **86**, 116–130 (2015)
47. T. Chen, Y.C. Wang, M.C. Chiu, A type-II fuzzy collaborative forecasting approach for productivity forecasting under an uncertainty environment. J. Ambient. Intell. Humaniz. Comput. **12**, 2751–2763 (2021)
48. T. Senapati, R.R. Yager, Fermatean fuzzy sets. J. Ambient. Intell. Humaniz. Comput. **11**, 663–674 (2020)
49. Y.C. Wang, H.R. Tsai, T. Chen, A selectively fuzzified back propagation network approach for precisely estimating the cycle time range in wafer fabrication. Mathematics **9**(12), 1430 (2021)
50. Y. Song, Q. Fu, Y.F. Wang, X. Wang, Divergence-based cross entropy and uncertainty measures of Atanassov's intuitionistic fuzzy sets with their application in decision making. Appl. Soft Comput. **84**, 105703 (2019)
51. T. Chen, A FAHP-FTOPSIS approach for choosing mid-term occupational healthcare measures amid the COVID-19 pandemic. Health Policy Technol. **10**(2), 100517 (2021)
52. J. Ye, J. Zhan, W. Ding, H. Fujita, A novel fuzzy rough set model with fuzzy neighborhood operators. Inf. Sci. **544**, 266–297 (2021)
53. T.C.T. Chen, C.W. Lin, Assessing cloud manufacturing applications using an optimally rectified FAHP approach. Compl. Intell. Syst. **8**(6), 5087–5099 (2022)
54. R.M. Rodríguez, L. Martínez, V. Torra, Z.S. Xu, F. Herrera, Hesitant fuzzy sets: state of the art and future directions. Int. J. Intell. Syst. **29**(6), 495–524 (2014)
55. G. Büyüközkan, E. Mukul, Evaluation of smart health technologies with hesitant fuzzy linguistic MCDM methods. J. Intell. Fuzzy Syst. **39**(5), 6363–6375 (2020)
56. T.C.T. Chen, H.C. Wu, A partial-consensus and unequal-authority fuzzy collaborative intelligence approach for assessing robotic applications amid the COVID-19 pandemic. Soft. Comput. **27**(22), 16493–16509 (2023)
57. A. Moral, C. Castiello, L. Magdalena, C. Mencar, *Explainable Fuzzy Systems* (Springer International Publishing, 2021)
58. T.C.T. Chen, in *Explainable Artificial Intelligence (XAI) in Manufacturing: Methodology, Tools, and Applications*. Applications of XAI for Forecasting in the Manufacturing Domain (2023), pp. 13–50
59. M. T. Ribeiro, S. Singh, C. Guestrin, in *Proceedings of the 22nd ACM SIGKDD International Conference on Knowledge Discovery and Data Mining*. "Why Should I Trust You?" Explaining the Predictions of Any Classifier (2016), pp. 1135–1144
60. Y.C. Wang, T. Chen, Adapted techniques of explainable artificial intelligence for explaining genetic algorithms on the example of job scheduling. Expert Syst. Appl. 121369 (2023)
61. T. Chen, Y.C. Wang, A modified random forest incremental interpretation method for explaining artificial and deep neural networks in cycle time prediction. Decis. Anal. J. **7**, 100226 (2023)
62. E. Ogasawara, L.C. Martinez, D. De Oliveira, G. Zimbrão, G.L., Pappa, M. Mattoso, in *The 2010 International Joint Conference on Neural Networks*. Adaptive Normalization: A Novel Data Normalization Approach for Non-stationary Time Series (2010), pp. 1–8
63. Y.C. Wang, T. Chen, M.-C. Chiu, An improved explainable artificial intelligence tool in healthcare for hospital recommendation. Healthcare Anal. **3**, 100147 (2023)
64. B. Mahbooba, M. Timilsina, R. Sahal, M. Serrano, Explainable artificial intelligence (XAI) to enhance trust management in intrusion detection systems using decision tree model. Complexity **2021**, 6634811 (2021)

65. H.C. Wu, T.C.T. Chen, M.C. Chiu, Assessing the sustainability of smart healthcare applications using a multi-perspective fuzzy comprehensive evaluation approach. Digital Health **9**, 20552076231203904 (2023)
66. T.C.T. Chen, in *Explainable Artificial Intelligence (XAI) in Manufacturing: Methodology, Tools, and Applications.* Applications of XAI for Decision Making in the Manufacturing Domain (2023), pp. 51–81
67. B. Gulowaty, M. Woźniak, in *2021 International Joint Conference on Neural Networks.* Extracting Interpretable Decision Tree Ensemble from Random Forest (2021), pp. 1–8
68. T.C.T. Chen, Applications of XAI to job sequencing and scheduling in manufacturing. in *Explainable Artificial Intelligence (XAI) in Manufacturing: Methodology, Tools, and Applications* (2023), pp. 83–105
69. J.M. Mendel, P.P. Bonissone, Critical thinking about explainable AI (XAI) for rule-based fuzzy systems. IEEE Trans. Fuzzy Syst. **29**(12), 3579–3593 (2021)
70. T.C.T. Chen, in *Sustainable Smart Healthcare: Lessons Learned from the COVID-19 Pandemic.* Evaluating the Sustainability of a Smart Healthcare Application (2023), pp. 39–63
71. M.S. Islam, M.A. Awal, J.N. Laboni, F.T. Pinki, S. Karmokar, K.M. Mumenin, S. Al-Ahmadi, Md.A. Rahman, Md.S. Hossain, S. Mirjalili, HGSORF: Henry gas solubility optimization-based random forest for c-section prediction and XAI-based cause analysis. Comput. Biol. Med. **147**, 105671 (2022)
72. Y.C. Wang, T. Chen, M.C. Chiu, An explainable deep-learning approach for job cycle time prediction. Decis. Anal. J. **6**, 100153 (2023)
73. T.C.T. Chen, in *Explainable Artificial Intelligence (XAI) in Manufacturing: Methodology, Tools, and Applications.* Explainable Artificial Intelligence (XAI) in Manufacturing (2023), pp. 1–11
74. Y.-C. Wang, T. Chen, Y.-C. Lin, 3D printer selection for aircraft component manufacturing using a nonlinear FGM and dependency-considered fuzzy VIKOR approach. Aerospace **10**, 591 (2023)
75. D. Karaboga, E. Kaya, Adaptive network based fuzzy inference system (ANFIS) training approaches: a comprehensive survey. Artif. Intell. Rev. **52**, 2263–2293 (2019)
76. T.C.T. Chen, C.W. Lin, M.C. Chiu, Optimizing 3D printing facility selection for ubiquitous manufacturing using an evolving fuzzy big data analytics approach. Int. J. Adv. Manuf. Technol. **127**, 4111–4121 (2023)
77. A.L. Buczak, C.M. Gifford, in *ACM SIGKDD Workshop on Intelligence and Security Informatics.* Fuzzy Association Rule Mining for Community Crime Pattern Discovery (2010), pp. 1–10
78. T.C.T. Chen, Y.C. Wang, M.C. Chiu, An efficient approximating alpha-cut operations approach for deriving fuzzy priorities in fuzzy multi-criterion decision-making. Appl. Soft Comput. **139**, 110238 (2023)
79. H.C. Wu, H.R. Tsai, T.C.T. Chen, K.W. Hsu, Energy-efficient production planning using a two-stage fuzzy approach. Mathematics **9**(10), 1101 (2021)
80. T. Chen, C.W. Lin, Y.C. Wang, An auto-weighting FWI fuzzy collaborative intelligence approach for forecasting DRAM yield. Proc. Manuf. **55**, 102–109 (2021)
81. H. Moayedi, M. Raftari, A. Sharifi, W.A.W. Jusoh, A.S.A. Rashid, Optimization of ANFIS with GA and PSO estimating α ratio in driven piles. Eng. Comput. **36**, 227–238 (2020)
82. M.C. Chiu, T.C.T. Chen, K.W. Hsu, Modeling an uncertain productivity learning process using an interval fuzzy methodology. Mathematics **8**(6), 998 (2020)
83. T. Chen, M.C. Chiu, An interval fuzzy number-based fuzzy collaborative forecasting approach for DRAM yield forecasting. Compl. Intell. Syst. **7**, 111–122 (2021)

Chapter 4
XAmI Applications to Location-Aware Services

Abstract Location-aware (or location-based) services (LASs) are probably the most prevalent application of ambient intelligence (AmI). This chapter first summarizes the applications of artificial intelligence (AI) in LASs. However, some AI applications in LASs are difficult to understand or communicate with mobile users, so explainable ambient intelligence (XAmI) techniques must be applied to enhance the understandability of such AI applications. To this end, some XAmI techniques for LASs have been introduced. Subsequently, various types of interpretations of LASs are explained through examples. In addition, the priorities and impacts of criteria for choosing suitable service locations are also distinguished. Furthermore, to enhance the interpretability of the recommendation process and result for users, visualization XAmI methods tailored for LASs are also reviewed. This section concludes with a discussion of how to interpret AI-based optimization in LASs.

Keywords Location-aware service · Explainable artificial intelligence · Visualization · Recommendation

4.1 Artificial Intelligence (AI) Applications in Location-Aware Services (LASs)

Location-aware services (LASs) are a major application field of ambient intelligence (AmI) [1]. As in other fields of AmI, artificial intelligence (AI) technologies have been widely used in LASs [2–3]. Some applications are easy for users to understand. For example, Chen [1] proposed a fuzzy mixed integer-nonlinear programming (FMINLP) model to identify the most suitable fast food chain to serve customers in a timely manner, where fuzzy logic was used to model uncertainty in meal preparation times and user travel times [4–5]. Ordinary fuzzy logic basically requires no explanation. Fuzzy rules, that is, decision rules with linguistic terms, are even widely used to explain the reasoning mechanisms of many complex AI applications [6–7]. In addition, mathematical programming models may be difficult to optimize [8–9], but are easy to understand for planners and users.

© The Author(s), under exclusive license to Springer Nature Switzerland AG 2024
T.-C. T. Chen, *Explainable Ambient Intelligence (XAmI)*,
SpringerBriefs in Applied Sciences and Technology,
https://doi.org/10.1007/978-3-031-54935-9_4

   Some AI applications to LASs are even more complicated, involving artificial neural networks (ANN), deep learning, advanced fuzzy logic, stochastic methods, etc. For example, Vukovic et al. [10] predicted user movement in the context of enhanced location-aware services, for which a three-layer feedforward network (FNN) [11] was constructed. The FNN read a user's two subsequent movements and predicted his/her next movement. In order to provide visitors with a better museum visiting experience, Tsai et al. [12] built a backpropagation network (BPN) [13–14] to detect the location of each visitor based on the signal emitted by his/her handheld device. Lin and Chen [15] proposed a type-II fuzzy method to help travelers choose suitable travel destinations during the COVID-19 pandemic, in which the fuzzy analytic hierarchy process (FAHP) [16–17] was applied to derive the priorities of criteria for making such choices. The type-II fuzzy vise kriterijumska optimizacija i kompromisno resenje (VIKOR) method [18] was devised to rank the overall performances of possible travel destinations.

   Yin et al. [19] is an application of collaborative filtering (CF) technique in LAS. Users with similar conditions were grouped and recommended similar services (or service locations), for which the most critical condition was location. The recommendation results were verified through user feedback (including the quality of service) [20]. Only quality services were recommended to future users. However, sometimes users did not give feedback on the quality of their services. Yin et al. assumed a distribution of the quality of service and derived the parameters of the distributions. Although stochastic prediction is considered a highly interpretable artificial intelligence model [21], stochastic methods with unknown distributions are far from being accepted and understood.

   Sarker et al. [22] discussed the application of decision trees (DTs) in predicting mobile user behavior. They highlighted the problem of overfitting due to the large number of leaves (outcomes) generated in a DT. However, there was no such change in user behavior. To address this issue, Sarker et al. considered context-aware issues when splitting nodes to generate leaves. In this way, the number of possible leaves was greatly reduced. One advantage of their proposed methodology is that DTs are a naturally understandable AI method that requires no explanation [23]. However, DTs may not be accurate enough, which is one of the disadvantages.

   Kumar and Singh [24] mined the text messages left by a user on his/her Twitter account to identify the user's location during emergencies. To this end, a deep learning method [25], a convolutional neural network (CNN), was constructed and optimized. CNN is a well-known AI method for natural language processing. CNN is also very effective in image or pattern recognition [26]. However, CNNs are also known for their low understandability and communicability.

4.2 Issues of Existing AI Applications in LASs

According to Tsai and Chen [27], existing LASs have the following issues:

- There is no systematic procedure for designing practical LASs.
- Most LAS applications have not conducted cost–benefit analyses. One reason is that large-scale government support is not for profit. Another reason is that it is difficult to collect client/user-related information. Additionally, linking the user's final operation with the service provided by a LAS is a difficult task. However, to ensure the sustainability of a LAS, these must be overcome to enable a reliable cost–benefit analysis.
- Most LASs are not always durable; therefore, the continued development of new LASs may not be worthwhile.
- Most LAS applications can be modeled as human–computer interaction processes, in which human factors/Ergonomics are an integral part and should be taken seriously.

LAS systems can solve their problems and pursue sustainable development in the following ways [27]: continuously updating the database, adding new functions and eliminating uninteresting services, providing more choices and flexibility, and improving the suitability of use. This involves many aspects and is a process that relies heavily on user feedback and must evolve over time [28] (see Fig. 4.1). In addition, this process can be considered as a long-term optimization process, and some small-scale short-term optimization actions will be taken at each point in time to improve the LAS system. However, since the smooth operation of a LAS system is a very difficult task, most LAS systems are not yet optimized. One possible reason is that some LAS systems must serve many people simultaneously. Even in the short term, the problem of optimizing the performance of a LAS for multiple users is extremely complex [29]. Furthermore, LASs aim to meet the diverse and time-varying needs of users, which cannot be fully quantified.

A characteristic of these applications is that the users of LASs are ordinary people from every possible background, without any specific knowledge [30–31]. Therefore, most AI technologies applied to LASs may be difficult for them to understand, making the application of explainable ambient intelligence (XAmI) imperative [32–35].

4.3 XAmI Applications in Location-Aware Services

4.3.1 Suitable XAmI Methods for Location-Aware Services

Existing XAmI methods can be divided into three categories: pre-model XAmI methods, intrinsic XAmI methods, and post-model XAmI methods [36] (see Fig. 4.2):

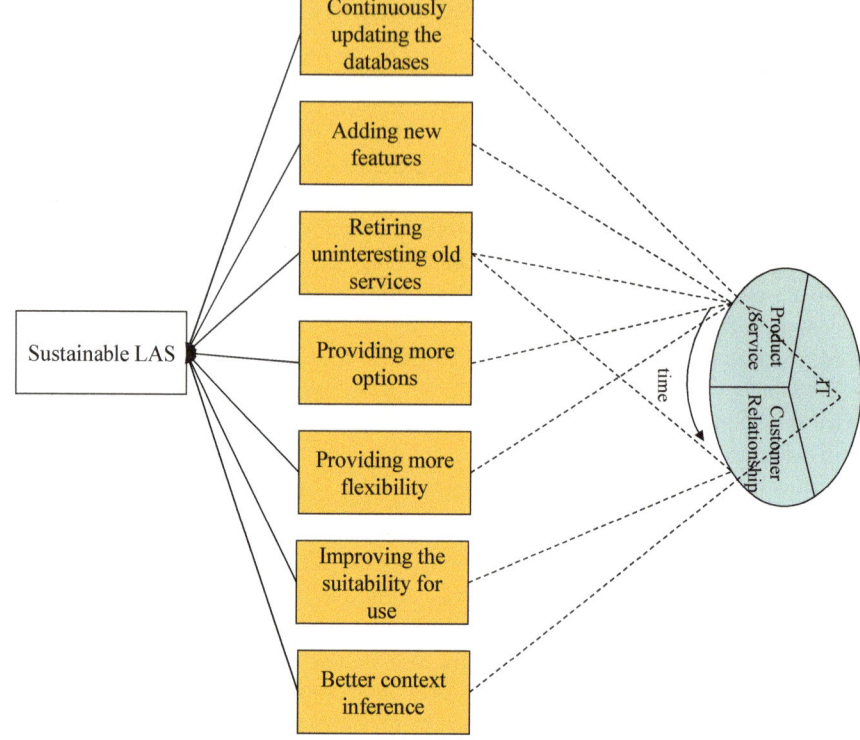

Fig. 4.1 Toward a sustainable LAS

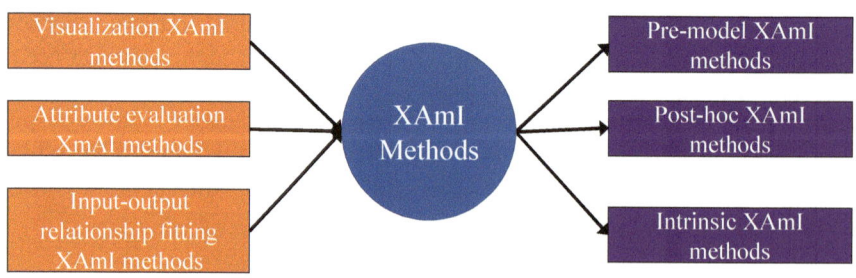

Fig. 4.2 Classification of XAmI methods

- **Pre-model XAmI methods**: Pre-model XAmI methods focus on the analysis of input data, which is especially important for XAmI applications to capture users' conditions and requirements in LASs. For example, a restaurant recommendation system might discover that most users in a certain area are students during lunchtime because there is a university in the area (see Fig. 4.3). Figure 4.3, a box-and-whisker plot showing user age distribution, is a prevalent pre-model XAmI method. In addition to user data, service location information is an important input to a LAS and therefore needs to be analyzed. For example, in Lin and Chen [15], in order to recommend appropriate COVID-19 vaccination sites to users, the expected waiting time at COVID-19 vaccination sites as well as the crowding and reliability of vaccination sites were estimated.

- **Post hoc XAmI methods**: In contrast, the criteria for selecting an appropriate service (or service location) are usually specified by the user. Therefore, post hoc XAmI methods are of little use. Or, in other words, the application of post hoc XAmI methods focuses on deriving the priorities of criteria if the user does not explicitly state them or only gives approximate relative priorities [9]. Additionally, sometimes users may not know what they actually care about when making a choice. There are some LASs that try to solve this problem by estimating the importance of such hidden criteria by comparing the recommendation results with users' choices [37].

- **Intrinsic XAmI methods**: Intrinsic XAmI methods aim to fit the relationship between the input and output of an AI application. In this respect, inference mechanisms in LASs are often simpler than those in AI applications in other fields. ANNs or deep learning, which are difficult to understand, are less commonly used in LASs. In comparison, easier-to-understand multi-criteria decision-making methods, such as the technique for order preference by similarity to ideal solution (TOPSIS) [38–39], and VIKOR, are more common. Fuzzy ordered weighted average (OWA) and its variants are also frequently applied for service (or service location) recommendation in LASs, some of which are very complex and difficult to understand due to the incorporation of advanced fuzzy sets [40–41]. One trend to address this problem is interpretable fuzzy logic, which aims to explain the reasoning processes in such complex applications with less advanced fuzzy sets (or rules) or even crisp sets (and rules) [42–43].

Another classification divides existing XAmI methods into the following categories (see Fig. 4.2) [7]:

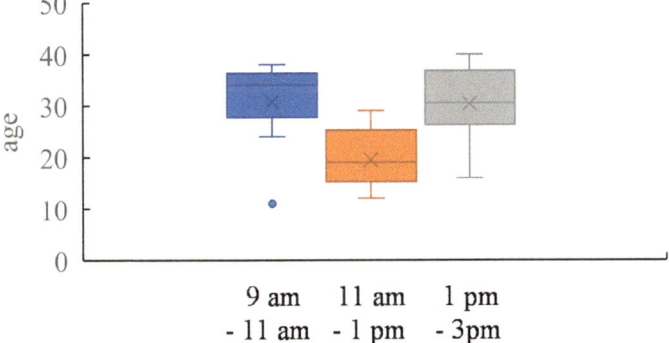

Fig. 4.3 Box-and-whisker plot showing user age distribution

- **Visualization XAmI methods**: XAmI techniques and tools for visualizing operations in the AI application.
- **Attribute evaluation XAmI methods**: XAmI techniques and tools for evaluating the effect, contribution, or importance of each input on the output.
- **Input–output relationship fitting XAmI methods**: XAmI techniques and tools for approximating the relationship between the inputs and output of the AI application.

This classification is similar to the previous classification, except that the first category emphasizes the use of visual tools to enhance user understanding.

4.3.2   Various Types of Explanations for Location-Aware Services

There are multiple types of explanations for the AI application of a LAS. For example, a **global explanation** of an AI application can be

- the system architecture diagram of the AI application,
- a text description, flowchart, or pseudocode describing the algorithm's reasoning process,
- a snapshot of the user interface, and most importantly,
- the overall performance of the LAS.

System architecture diagrams of AI applications to LASs are usually combined with flowcharts [19, 44].

The overall performance of a LAS is usually evaluated in terms of the successful recommendation rate (s) [18, 45]:

$$s = \frac{1}{n} \sum_{i=1}^{n} I_i \tag{4.1}$$

$$I_i = \begin{cases} 1 & \text{if user } i \text{ followed the recommendation} \\ 0 & \text{otherwise} \end{cases} \tag{4.2}$$

Most LASs recommend the best-performing alternative to the user, who then selects one from among all alternatives. The successful recommendation rate is sufficient to consider this situation. However, in some cases, the user requires multiple recommendations, and the LAS will act accordingly, for example, recommending multiple nearby tourist spots to the traveler to visit, which performance can be evaluated by the $F1$ metric [46]:

$$F1 = \frac{2 \cdot \text{recall rate} \cdot \text{precision}}{\text{recall rate} + \text{precision}} \tag{4.3}$$

where

$$recall\ rate = \frac{|\mathbf{A} \cap \mathbf{R}|}{|\mathbf{A}|} \tag{4.4}$$

$$precision = \frac{|\mathbf{A} \cap \mathbf{R}|}{|\mathbf{R}|} \tag{4.5}$$

A and **R** represent the action set and recommendation set, respectively.

A **local interpretation** of a LAS tells a user how his/her recommendation was made [47–48], for example, for user k:

> If criterion #2 is slightly more important than criterion #1 and criterion #3 is considerably more important than criterion #1 and ... then service location A is recommended.

A **contrastive explanation** explains why one service location was recommended over another [49]. For example, for user k,

> Service location B was recommended because the estimated waiting time is (or must be) shorter than 30 min. If the estimated waiting time is (or may be) longer than 30 min, service location D is recommended instead.

In this regard, the **local foil method** [36] finds the minimal changes needed to change to a different recommendation.

Example 4.1 A hotel recommendation system recommended Hotel B to a user, and the user wanted to know why Hotel A was not recommended. A contrastive explanation is therefore required. The improvement that Hotel A should make to the performance of each criterion for it to be recommended is shown in Table 4.1. In this case, the required contrastive explanation is

> The reason why Hotel B is recommended instead of Hotel A is because Hotel A's performance is only 4 points when optimizing criterion #4. If that performance can be improved to 5 points, Hotel A will be recommended instead.

A contrastive explanation is also a special type of **what-if explanation**. Since LAS applications often involve heterogeneous types of data [19], **contingency table analysis** (or **cross-tabulation**) can also be applied to provide contrastive explanations (see Table 4.2).

Table 4.1 Improvement that Hotel A should make to the performance of each criterion

Criterion #	Original performance	Improved performance	%	Recommended hotel
1	2	3	50	B → A
2	3	4	33	B → A
3	1	3	200	B → A
4	4	5	25	B → A
5	3	5	67	B → A

Table 4.2 Contrastive explanation using contingency table analysis

Feature	Category	Number	Recommendation
Gender	Male	23	Hotel A, ...
	Female	24	Hotel B, ...
Age	20–30	13	Hotel B, ...
	30–40	25	Hotel A, ...
	>40	9	Hotel C, ...

4.3.3   Visualization XAmI Methods for Location-Aware Services

Location-based recommendation is one of the mainstreams of LAS. Many studies treated location-based recommendation as a multi-criteria decision-making problem, where the system compared alternatives that were close to a user based on the user's preferences in multiple aspects.

Lin and Chen [15] established a travel destination recommendation system, in which each traveler of a travel group compares the relative priorities of criteria for choosing a travel destination in pairs. The results by traveler k are placed into $\tilde{\mathbf{A}}(k)$, which can be visualized using **a gradient bar chart** in Fig. 4.4, in which the gradient bars illustrate the uncertainty of the membership functions (Fig. 4.5) [23, 50–51].

The fuzzy priorities of criteria can be derived by solving the following equations [52–54]:

$$\det(\tilde{\mathbf{A}}(k)(-)\tilde{\lambda}(k)\mathbf{I}) = 0 \qquad (4.6)$$

$$(\tilde{\mathbf{A}}(k)(-)\tilde{\lambda}(k))(\times)\tilde{\mathbf{x}}(k) = 0 \qquad (4.7)$$

Fig. 4.4 Gradient bar chart for visualizing pairwise comparison results

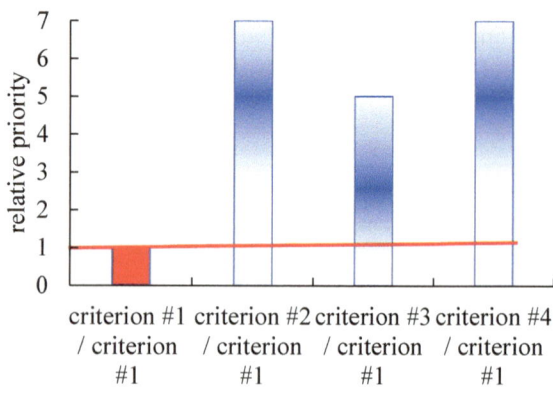

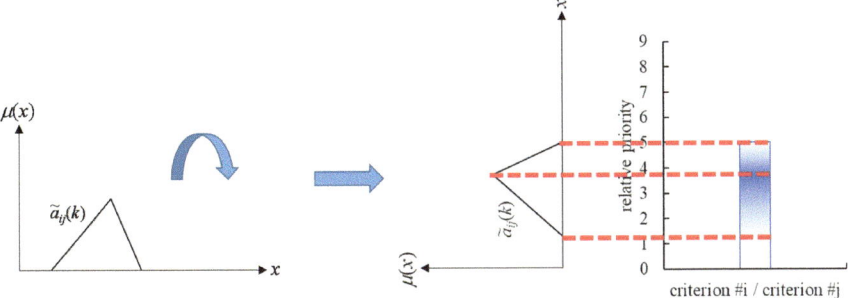

Fig. 4.5 Gradient bar for illustrating the uncertainty of the membership function

$$\tilde{w}_i(k) = \frac{\tilde{x}_i(k)}{\sum_{j=1}^{n} \tilde{x}_j(k)} \qquad (4.8)$$

$\tilde{\lambda}(k)$ and $\tilde{\mathbf{x}}(k)$ are the fuzzy eigenvalue and eigenvector of $\tilde{\mathbf{A}}(k)$, respectively. $\tilde{w}_i(k)$ is the fuzzy priority of criterion i to traveler k. Many methods, such as fuzzy geometric mean (FGM) [55–56], fuzzy extent analysis (FEA) [57], and alpha-cut operations (ACO) [58–59], can be applied to solve these equations. Lin and Chen [15] applied ACO to derive the fuzzy priorities of criteria, so the derivation results were not triangular fuzzy numbers (TFNs) anymore.

The fuzzy priorities can be illustrated using a line chart (Fig. 4.6). The line chart can be improved by applying the following XAmI techniques:

- **The common expression technique**: Technical terms and variable names should be replaced with common expressions.
- **The annotated figure technique**: The legend of each object should be placed close to the object.

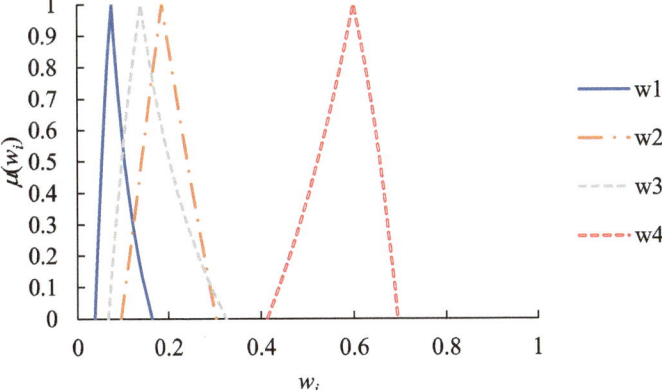

Fig. 4.6 Line chart for visualizing the derivation results

Fig. 4.7 Improved line chart

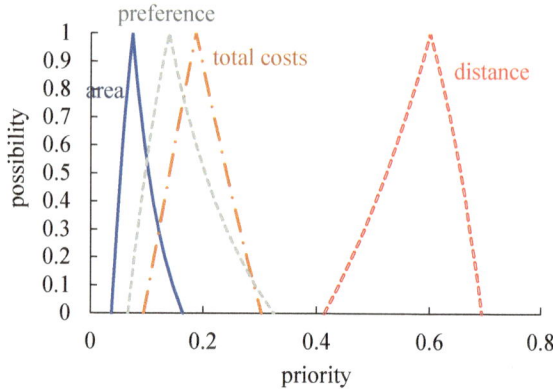

The results are shown in Fig. 4.7.

The derivation results can also be illustrated using a gradient bar chart, as shown in Fig. 4.8. Wang and Chen [35] validated the derivation results using another XAmI tool, a manually adjustable gradient bar chart, as shown in Fig. 4.9. The decision-maker can manually adjust the fuzzy priority of a criterion if the derivation result is unacceptable. However, raising the priority of one criterion will automatically lower the priorities of other criteria and vice versa.

Subsequently, the fuzzy priorities derived by all travelers are aggregated into a type-II fuzzy set, which can be illustrated using a line chart as well (Fig. 4.10):

$$\text{LMF} = \widetilde{FI}(\{\tilde{w}_i(k)|k = 1 \sim K\}) \tag{4.9}$$

$$\text{UMF} = \widetilde{\text{PCFI}}^{H/K}(\{\tilde{w}_i(k)|k = 1 \sim K\}) \tag{4.10}$$

where LMF and UMF denote the lower and upper membership functions of the aggregation result (i.e., a type-II fuzzy set), respectively. FI and PCFI indicate the

Fig. 4.8 Gradient bar chart for visualizing the derivation results

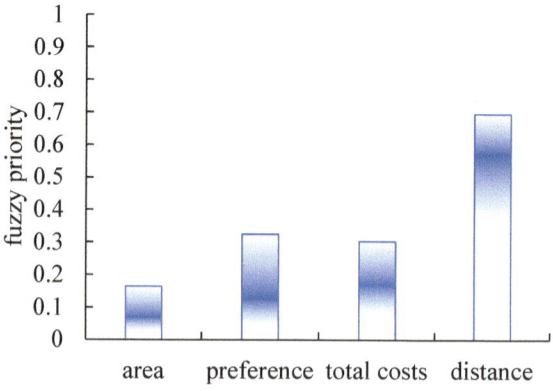

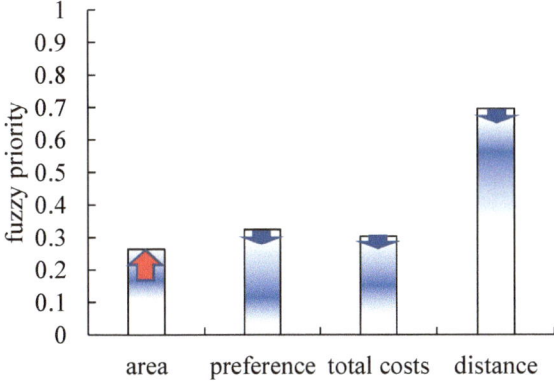

Fig. 4.9 Manually adjustable gradient bar chart to validate the derivation results

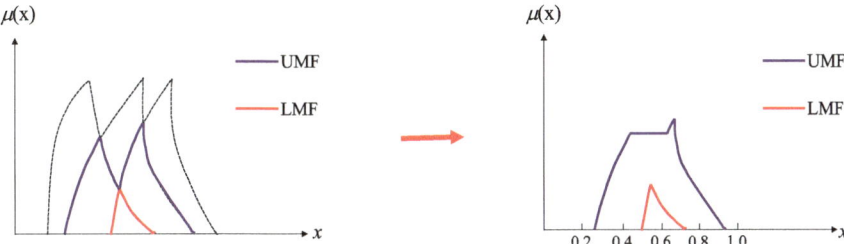

Fig. 4.10 Line chart for illustrating the aggregation process and result

fuzzy intersection and partial-consensus fuzzy intersection functions, respectively:

$$\mu_{\widetilde{FI}(\{\tilde{w}_i(k)|k=1\sim K\})}(x) = \min_k (\mu_{\tilde{w}_i(k)}(x)) \tag{4.11}$$

$$\mu_{\widetilde{PCFI}^{H/K}}(x) = \max_{\text{all } g}(\min(\mu_{\tilde{w}_1(g(1))}(x), \ldots, \mu_{\tilde{w}_1(g(H))}(x))) \tag{4.12}$$

where $g() \in Z^+$; $1 \le g() \le K$; $g(p) \cap g(q) = \emptyset \ \forall \ p \ne q$; $H \ge 2$.

The UMF is modified by connecting the disjointed intervals to facilitate the subsequent operations.

A traceable aggregation diagram (Fig. 4.11), which is another XAmI tools proposed by them, can be plotted to enhance the traceability of the aggregation result, which is essential to the interpretability:

- **Traceable aggregation diagram**: Simultaneously presenting the original data and aggregation result contributes to its credibility.

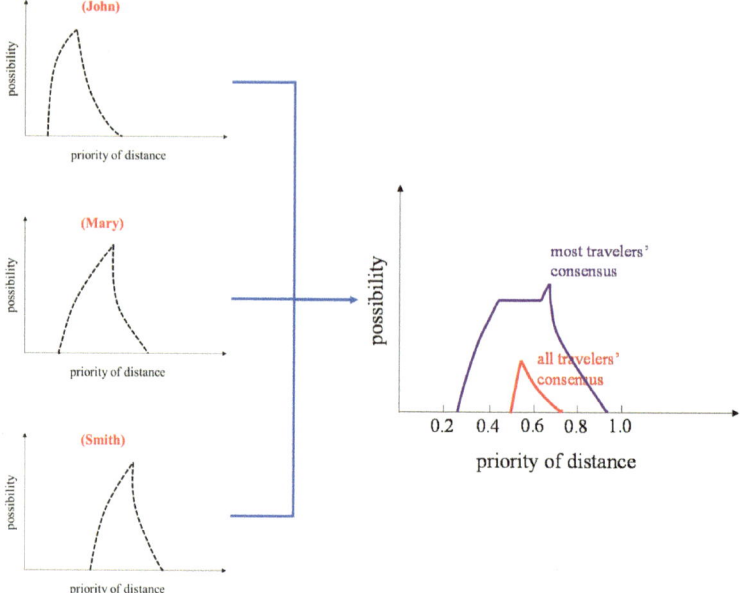

Fig. 4.11 Traceable aggregation diagram

Subsequently, a type-II fuzzy VIKOR method [62] is applied to evaluate the overall performance of a travel destination, which comprises the following steps.

Step 1. Determine the ideal performance in optimizing each criterion:

$$\tilde{p}_i^* = \max_h \tilde{p}_{hi} \tag{4.13}$$

$\tilde{p}_{hi}$ is the performance of alternative h in optimizing criterion i.

Step 2. Compute the normalized fuzzy distance from the ideal performance [63]:

$$\tilde{d}_{hi} = \frac{\tilde{p}_i^*(-)\tilde{p}_{hi}}{p_{i3}^* - \min_i(p_{i1})} \tag{4.14}$$

Step 3. Derive $\tilde{S}_h$ and $\tilde{R}_h$, both of which are type-II fuzzy sets [62]:

$$\tilde{S}_h = \sum_{i=1}^n (\tilde{w}_i(all)(\times)\tilde{d}_{hi}) \tag{4.15}$$

$$\tilde{R}_h = \max_i (\tilde{w}_i(all)(\times)\tilde{d}_{hi}) \tag{4.16}$$

$\tilde{S}_h$ and $\tilde{R}_h$ measure the average and worst ineffectiveness, respectively. Both are the smaller the better.

Step 4. Combine $\tilde{S}_h$ and $\tilde{R}_h$ into $\tilde{Q}_h$ as follows [62]:

$$
\begin{aligned}
\tilde{Q}_h &= \omega N(\tilde{S}_h)(+)(1-\omega)N(\tilde{R}_h) \\
&= \omega \cdot \frac{\tilde{S}_h(-)\min_r \tilde{S}_r}{\max(\max_r \tilde{S}_r) - \min(\min_r \tilde{S}_r)}(+)(1-\omega) \\
&\quad \cdot \frac{\tilde{R}_h(-)\min_r \tilde{R}_r}{\max(\max_r \tilde{R}_r) - \min(\min_r \tilde{R}_r)}
\end{aligned}
\tag{4.17}
$$

Just like $\tilde{S}_h$ and $\tilde{R}_h$, $\tilde{Q}_h$ is also the smaller the better.

Step 5. Defuzzify $\tilde{Q}_h$ using the center-of-gravity method [63], for which the weights of the LMF and UMF are set to ξ and $1 - \xi$, respectively [64]:

$$
\begin{aligned}
D(\tilde{Q}_h) &= (1 - \xi) \cdot \frac{\sum_\alpha \alpha \left(\frac{Q_{hu}^L(\alpha) + Q_{hu}^R(\alpha)}{2} \right)}{\sum_\alpha \alpha} \\
&\quad + \xi \cdot \frac{\sum_\alpha \alpha \left(\frac{Q_{hl}^L(\alpha) + Q_{hl}^R(\alpha)}{2} \right)}{\sum_\alpha \alpha}
\end{aligned}
\tag{4.18}
$$

By increasing the value of ξ, the overall consensus among all travelers becomes more important than the partial consensus among most travelers.

Step 6. Recommend the travel destination that achieved the highest $D(\tilde{Q}_h)$ value to the traveler group.

Lin and Chen [15] designed a new XAmI tool, the **segmented distance diagram**, to present the differences in the distances of alternatives from the ideal solution, so as to enhance the explainability of fuzzy VIKOR, as illustrated in Fig. 4.12:

- All possible alternatives surround the ideal solution.
- The distance between an alternative and the ideal solution is $\tilde{Q}_h$ composed of two segments: the longest distance $((1 - \omega)N(\tilde{R}_h))$ and overall distance $(\omega N(\tilde{S}_h))$ indicated with red and blue lines, respectively.

For example, in Fig. 4.11, alternative #2 is the best choice because it is closest to the ideal solution. In addition, the advantage of alternative #2 over other alternatives is that its overall distance is much shorter than other alternatives.

A non-recommended service (or service location) can improve its performance in optimizing various criteria, as shown in the following example.

Example 4.2 Lin and Chen [15] proposed a type-II fuzzy approach with XAmI for nature-based leisure travel destination selection amid the COVID-19 pandemic, in which a type-II fuzzy VIKOR method was applied to evaluate and compare the overall performances of possible travel destinations in Table 4.3. According to this

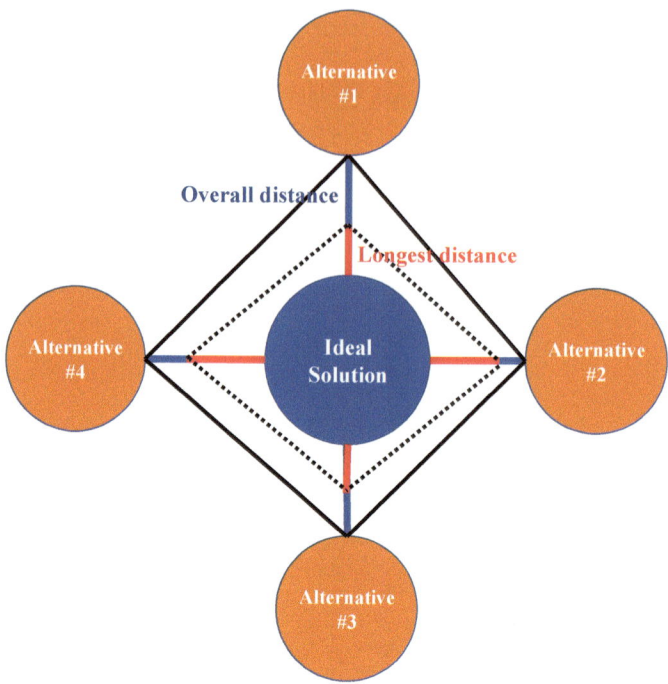

Fig. 4.12 Segmented distance diagram

table, Destination #4 was recommended to the travel group. Destination #2 ranked last. However, it is still possible to elevate the ranking of Destination #2 by improving its performances in optimizing various criteria. For example,

Table 4.3 Overall performances of possible nature-based leisure travel destinations

h	$D(\tilde{Q}_h)$	Ranking
1	0.276	2
2	0.566	5
3	0.436	4
4	0.066	1
5	0.281	3

Table 4.4 Updated overall performances of destinations

h	$D(\tilde{Q}_h)$	Ranking
1	0.291	3
2	0.072	1
3	0.483	5
4	0.088	2
5	0.294	4

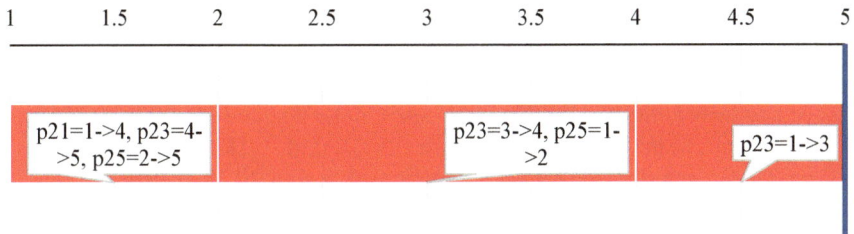

Fig. 4.13 Improvement process

Destination #2: Ranking #5 → #4 if $\tilde{p}_{23} = 1 \rightarrow 3$.

Followed by another improvement that further elevates the ranking:

Destination #2: Ranking #4 → #2 if $\tilde{p}_{23} = 3 \rightarrow 4$ and $\tilde{p}_{25} = 1 \rightarrow 2$.

Destination #2 can even be recommended if $\tilde{p}_{21} = 1 \rightarrow 4$, $\tilde{p}_{23} = 4 \rightarrow 5$, and $\tilde{p}_{25} = 2 \rightarrow 5$. The updated overall performances of destinations are shown in Table 4.4. The improvement process can be illustrated by a force plot (see Fig. 4.13), which is an XAmI tool usually used to compare the importance levels of features based on a SHAP analysis.

4.4 Criteria Priority Versus Impact

An important function of XAmI is to evaluate the impact of each input. However, from an XAmI perspective, higher priority criteria do not necessarily have a greater impact. The reason is that the performance in optimizing a criterion may already be the highest (or lowest) and therefore cannot be changed. Therefore, varying the performance does not change the overall performance, as shown in the example below.

Example 4.3 To help travelers choose suitable travel destinations during the COVID-19 pandemic, Lin and Chen [15] proposed a fuzzy approach, in which

Table 4.5 Impact of each input/criterion for travel destination #5

Criterion	Performance	+ 10	Change in Rank	− 10	Change in Rank
Number of confirmed cases	38	41.8	No change	34.2	No change
Distance	414 (min)	455.4	No change	372.6	No change
Preference	5	5[a]	No change	4.5	No change
Area	2787 (ha)	3065.7	No change	2508.3	No change
Total costs	700 (NTD)	770	No change	630	4 → 3

[a] Already maximum

FAHP was applied to derive the priorities of criteria for making such choices as

The number of confirmed COVID-19 cases in the region: (0.07, 0.15, 0.32).
The distance to the forest recreation area: (0.03, 0.06, 0.14).
The traveler's preference for the forest recreation area: (0.28, 0.49, 0.68).
Area (size): (0.03, 0.06, 0.13).
Total costs: (0.12, 0.25, 0.43).

"The traveler's preference for the forest recreation area" was the criterion with the highest priority. Five possible travel destinations were compared using fuzzy VIKOR. To evaluate the impact of each input (i.e., performance) for travel destination #5, the **partial derivation method** [7, 60-61] is applied by varying the performance in optimizing each criterion by 10%. The evaluation results are summarized in Table 4.5. Obviously, "total costs" is the criterion with the greatest impact on the rank of this travel destination, not "the traveler's preference for the forest recreation area."

4.5 Explaining AI-Based Optimization in LASs

4.5.1 Local and Contrastive Explanations for AI-Based Optimization in LASs

Optimization models are usually built in LASs to minimize users' costs and maximize their effectiveness and resource utilization. For example, Chen [66] built a ubiquitous clinic recommendation system for users who are on the move and may not be familiar with nearby areas and clinics. The uncertainty in the travel time from the user's location to each clinic was modeled using a fuzzy number, and a fuzzy mixed integer-nonlinear programming (FMINLP) model was then optimized to minimize the user's waiting time after arriving at the clinic. The FMINLP model was converted into a crisp mixed integer-nonlinear programming (MINLP) model and solved. The FIMNLP is far from easy to understand. Nevertheless, in the view of Wang and Chen [67]:

Table 4.6 Details of the optimization result to be conveyed to the user

Recommended Clinic	Route	Estimated Arrival time	Estimated Service Start Time
Clinic D	Go straight to Junction A, then turn left, go straight to Junction B, then turn right and go straight for 300 m	Approximately 6:30 PM	Around 6:45 PM

Table 4.7 Contrastive explanation of the optimization result

Comparison	Difference
Clinic D versus Clinic A	Preference for the doctor is the most important criterion. Preference for the doctor at Clinic D is 5, while preference for the doctor at Clinic A is only 3

- For most users, the optimization result will be much more important than the process. In fact, they don't care about the solution process.
- Users know that the optimal solution satisfies all constraints, but they are not sure how much the optimal solution is better than other solutions.

Therefore, each user should be provided with the following **local explanation** (Table 4.6):

- The optimal solution and its performance: For example, in a clinic recommendation system, a user should be provided with the clinic that is most suitable for the user and the relevant routes to the clinic to minimize the waiting time. Users who arrive at the clinic too early or too late may have to wait.
- The estimated time for the user to arrive at the service location: The arrival time can be represented by a fuzzy value $\tilde{v} = (v_1, v_2, v_3)$ derived from the optimization model to reflect its uncertainty. Furthermore, the derivation result can be conveyed using linguistic terms (e.g., "about/approximately," "quickly," "friendly," "comfortable," etc.) as "the time to arrive at the clinic is approximately v_2 (or from v_1 to v_3)" [68].
- The estimated time when the user will start to be served: This time is also a fuzzy number, which can be described by something like "you will see doctors around s_2 (or between s_1 and s_3)."

The user may be interested in comparing the recommended service location with another service location that interests him/her. To this end, the LAS highlighted the largest differences between the performances of the two service locations (see Table 4.7) in terms of a **contrastive explanation**.

References

1. T. Chen, Creating a just-in-time location-aware service using fuzzy logic. Appl. Spat. Anal. Policy **26**(9), 287–307 (2016)
2. P. Grifoni, A. D'Ulizia, F. Ferri, in *Mobile Big Data: A Roadmap from Models to Technologies*. Context-Awareness in Location Based Services in the Big Data Era (2018), pp. 85–127
3. T. Chen, A fuzzy integer-nonlinear programming approach for creating a flexible just-in-time location-aware service in a mobile environment. Appl. Soft Comput. **38**, 805–816 (2016)
4. M.C. Chiu, T.C. Chen, K.W. Hsu, Modeling an uncertain productivity learning process using an interval fuzzy methodology. Mathematics **8**(6), 998 (2020)
5. T. Chen, Y.C. Wang, M.C. Chiu, A type-II fuzzy collaborative forecasting approach for productivity forecasting under an uncertainty environment. J. Ambient. Intell. Humaniz. Comput. **12**, 2751–2763 (2021)
6. J. van der Waa, E. Nieuwburg, A. Cremers, M. Neerincx, Evaluating XAI: a comparison of rule-based and example-based explanations. Artif. Intell. **291**, 103404 (2021)
7. T.C.T. Chen, in *Explainable Artificial Intelligence (XAI) in Manufacturing: Methodology, Tools, and Applications*. Applications of XAI for Forecasting in the Manufacturing Domain (2023), pp. 13–50
8. M. Rabbani, M. Aghabegloo, H. Farrokhi-Asl, Solving a bi-objective mathematical programming model for bloodmobiles location routing problem. Int. J. Ind. Eng. Comput. **8**(1), 19–32 (2017)
9. Y.C. Lin, T. Chen, L.C. Wang, Integer nonlinear programming and optimized weighted-average approach for mobile hotel recommendation by considering travelers' unknown preferences. Oper. Res. Int. J. **18**, 625–643 (2018)
10. M. Vukovic, I. Lovrek, D. Jevtic, in *2007 15th International Conference on Software, Telecommunications and Computer Networks*. Predicting User Movement for Advanced Location-Aware Services (2007), pp. 1–5
11. T. Chen, Y.C. Wang, A modified random forest incremental interpretation method for explaining artificial and deep neural networks in cycle time prediction. Decis. Anal. J. **7**, 100226 (2023)
12. C.Y. Tsai, S.Y. Chou, S.W. Lin, in *Collaborative Product and Service Life Cycle Management for a Sustainable World: Proceedings of the 15th ISPE International Conference on Concurrent Engineering*. Location-Aware Tour Guide Systems in Museum (2008), pp. 349–356
13. B. Oztaysi, S.C. Onar, C. Kahraman, in *11th Conference of the European Society for Fuzzy Logic and Technology*. Outlier Detection in Location Based Systems by Using Fuzzy Clustering (2019), pp. 653–659
14. Y.C. Wang, H.R. Tsai, T. Chen, A selectively fuzzified back propagation network approach for precisely estimating the cycle time range in wafer fabrication. Mathematics **9**(12), 1430 (2021)
15. Y.C. Lin, T.C.T. Chen, An intelligent system for assisting personalized COVID-19 vaccination location selection: Taiwan as an example. Digital Health **8**, 20552076221109064 (2022)
16. N.B. Salah, I.B. Saadi, in *IEEE Conferences on Ubiquitous Intelligence & Computing, Advanced and Trusted Computing, Scalable Computing and Communications, Cloud and Big Data Computing, Internet of People, and Smart World Congress*. Fuzzy AHP for Learning Service Selection in Context-Aware Ubiquitous Learning Systems (2016), pp. 171–179
17. T.C.T. Chen, C.W. Lin, Assessing cloud manufacturing applications using an optimally rectified FAHP approach. Compl. Intell. Syst. **8**(6), 5087–5099 (2022)
18. Y.-C. Wang, T. Chen, Y.-C. Lin, 3D printer selection for aircraft component manufacturing using a nonlinear FGM and dependency-considered fuzzy VIKOR approach. Aerospace **10**, 591 (2023)
19. Y. Yin, L. Chen, J. Wan, Location-aware service recommendation with enhanced probabilistic matrix factorization. IEEE Access **6**, 62815–62825 (2018)
20. Y.C. Wang, T. Chen, M.-C. Chiu, An improved explainable artificial intelligence tool in healthcare for hospital recommendation. Healthcare Anal. **3**, 100147 (2023)
21. M. McNamara, Explainable AI: what is it? How does it work? And what role does data play? (2022). https://www.netapp.com/blog/explainable-ai/

22. I.H. Sarker, A. Colman, J. Han, A.I. Khan, Y.B. Abushark, K. Salah, Behavdt: a behavioral decision tree learning to build user-centric context-aware predictive model. Mobile Netw. Appl. **25**, 1151–1161 (2020)
23. T.C.T. Chen, in *Explainable Artificial Intelligence (XAI) in Manufacturing: Methodology, Tools, and Applications.* Applications of XAI for Decision Making in the Manufacturing Domain (2023), pp. 51–81
24. E. Kaasinen, User needs for location-aware mobile services. Pers. Ubiquit. Comput. **7**(1), 70–79 (2003)
25. Y.C. Wang, T. Chen, M.C. Chiu, An explainable deep-learning approach for job cycle time prediction. Decis. Anal. J. **6**, 100153 (2023)
26. T.C.T. Chen, in *Production Planning and Control in Semiconductor Manufacturing: Big Data Analytics and Industry 4.0 Applications.* Defect Pattern Analysis, Yield Learning Modeling, and Yield Prediction (2023), pp. 63–76
27. H.R. Tsai, T. Chen, Enhancing the sustainability of a location-aware service through optimization. Sustainability **6**(12), 9441–9455 (2014)
28. T. Chen, C.-W. Lin, Optimizing 3D printing facility selection for ubiquitous manufacturing using an evolving fuzzy big data analytics approach. Int. J. Adv. Manuf. Technol. **127**, 4111–4121 (2023)
29. A. Al-Refaie, T. Chen, M. Judeh, Optimal operating room scheduling for normal and unexpected events in a smart hospital. Oper. Res. Int. J. **18**(3), 579–602 (2018)
30. A. Kumar, J.P. Singh, Location reference identification from tweets during emergencies: a deep learning approach. Int. J. Disaster Risk Reduct. **33**, 365–375 (2019)
31. Y.C. Wang, T.C.T. Chen, M.C. Chiu, A systematic approach to enhance the explainability of artificial intelligence in healthcare with application to diagnosis of diabetes. Healthcare Anal. **3**, 100183 (2023)
32. D. Gunning, M. Stefik, J. Choi, T. Miller, S. Stumpf, G.Z. Yang, XAI—explainable artificial intelligence. Sci. Rob. 4(37), eaay7120 (2019)
33. T.C.T. Chen, in *Explainable Artificial Intelligence (XAI) in Manufacturing: Methodology, Tools, and Applications.* Explainable Artificial Intelligence (XAI) in Manufacturing (2023), pp. 1–11
34. L. Sanneman, J.A. Shah, The situation awareness framework for explainable AI (SAFE-AI) and human factors considerations for XAI systems. Int. J. Human Comput. Interact. **38**(18–20), 1772–1788 (2022)
35. Y.C. Wang, T. Chen, New XAI tools for selecting suitable 3D printing facilities in ubiquitous manufacturing. Compl. Intell. Syst. 1–17 (2023)
36. U. Kamath, J. Liu, *Explainable Artificial Intelligence: An Introduction to Interpretable Machine Learning* (Springer, 2021)
37. T.C.T. Chen, Y.C. Wang, An incremental learning and integer-nonlinear programming approach to mining users' unknown preferences for ubiquitous hotel recommendation. J. Ambient. Intell. Humaniz. Comput. **10**, 2771–2780 (2019)
38. Y. Çelikbilek, F. Tüysüz, An in-depth review of theory of the TOPSIS method: an experimental analysis. J. Manage. Anal. **7**(2), 281–300 (2020)
39. T. Chen, Y.C. Wang, P.H. Jiang, A selectively calibrated derivation technique and generalized fuzzy TOPSIS for semiconductor supply chain localization assessment. Decis. Anal. J. **8**, 100275 (2023)
40. C., Kahraman, F. K., Gündoğdu, A., Karaşan, & E. Boltürk, in *Customer Oriented Product Design: Intelligent and Fuzzy Techniques.* Advanced Fuzzy Sets and Multicriteria Decision Making on Product Development (2020), pp. 283–302
41. T.C.T. Chen, in *Advances in Fuzzy Group Decision Making.* Introduction to Fuzzy Group Decision Making (2022), pp. 1–7
42. T. Rutkowski, K. Łapa, R. Nielek, On explainable fuzzy recommenders and their performance evaluation. Int. J. Appl. Math. Comput. Sci. **29**(3), 595–610 (2019)
43. T. Chen, Guaranteed-consensus posterior-aggregation fuzzy analytic hierarchy process method. Neural Comput. Appl. **32**, 7057–7068 (2020)

44. M.C. Chiu, T.C.T. Chen, A ubiquitous healthcare system of 3D printing facilities for making dentures: application of type-II fuzzy logic. Digital Health **8**, 20552076221092540 (2022)
45. M.-C. Chiu, T. Chen, Assessing sustainable effectiveness of the adjustment mechanism of a ubiquitous clinic recommendation system. Health Care Manag. Sci. **23**, 239–248 (2020)
46. F. Yu, Q. Liu, S. Wu, L. Wang, T. Tan, in *Proceedings of the 39th International ACM SIGIR conference on Research and Development in Information Retrieval*. A Dynamic Recurrent Model for Next Basket Recommendation (2016), pp. 729–732
47. T.C.T. Chen, in *Explainable Artificial Intelligence (XAI) in Manufacturing: Methodology, Tools, and Applications*. Applications of XAI to Job Sequencing and Scheduling in Manufacturing (2023), pp. 83–105
48. D. Nguyen, in *Proceedings of the 2018 Conference of the North American Chapter of the Association for Computational Linguistics: Human Language Technologies,* vol. 1. Comparing Automatic and Human Evaluation of Local Explanations for Text Classification (2018), pp. 1069–1078
49. T.C.T. Chen, in *Sustainable Smart Healthcare: Lessons Learned from the COVID-19 Pandemic*. Enhancing the Sustainability of Smart Healthcare Applications with XAI (2023), pp. 93–110
50. Y.-C. Lin, T. Chen, Type-II fuzzy approach with explainable artificial intelligence for nature-based leisure travel destination selection amid the COVID-19 pandemic. Digital Health **8**, 20552076221106320 (2022)
51. T.C.T. Chen, M.C. Chiu, Evaluating the sustainability of smart technology applications in healthcare after the COVID-19 pandemic: a hybridising subjective and objective fuzzy group decision-making approach with explainable artificial intelligence. Digital Health **8**, 20552076221136380 (2022)
52. D. Božanić, D. Pamučar, D. Bojanić, Modification of the analytic hierarchy process (AHP) method using fuzzy logic: Fuzzy AHP approach as a support to the decision making process concerning engagement of the group for additional hindering. Serb. J. Manage. **10**(2), 151–171 (2015)
53. T. Chen, A FAHP-FTOPSIS approach for choosing mid-term occupational healthcare measures amid the COVID-19 pandemic. Health Policy Technol. **10**(2), 100517 (2021)
54. H.C. Wu, Y.C. Lin, T.C.T. Chen, Leisure agricultural park selection for traveler groups amid the COVID-19 pandemic. Agriculture **12**(1), 111 (2022)
55. D. Ajay, S. Broumi, J. Aldring, An MCDM method under neutrosophic cubic fuzzy sets with geometric bonferroni mean operator. Neutrosoph. Sets Syst. **32**, 187–202 (2020)
56. T. Chen, Assessing factors critical to smart technology applications in mobile health care—the FGM-FAHP approach. Health Policy Technol. **9**, 194–203 (2020)
57. Y.-C. Wang, T. Chen, Y.-L. Yeh, Advanced 3D printing technologies for the aircraft industry: a fuzzy systematic approach for assessing the critical factors. Int. J. Adv. Manuf. Technol. **105**, 4059–4069 (2019)
58. M. Khodagholi, A. Dolati, A. Hoseinzadeh, The solving an inverse 1-median problem by using alpha-cut fuzzy. J. Decis. Oper. Res. **3**(1), 58–71 (2018)
59. T. Chen, Evaluating the sustainability of a smart technology application to mobile health care—the FGM-ACO-FWA approach. Compl. Intell. Syst. **6**, 109–121 (2020)
60. E. Zaitseva, V. Levashenko, J. Kostolny, in *2012 International Conference on Quality, Reliability, Risk, Maintenance, and Safety Engineering*. Multi-State System Importance Analysis Based on Direct Partial Logic Derivative (2012), pp. 1514–1519
61. T. Chen, Y.C. Lin, M.C. Chiu, Approximating alpha-cut operations approach for effective and efficient fuzzy analytic hierarchy process analysis. Appl. Soft Comput. **85**, 105855 (2019)
62. J. Qin, X. Liu, W. Pedrycz, An extended VIKOR method based on prospect theory for multiple attribute decision making under interval type-2 fuzzy environment. Knowl. Based Syst. **86**, 116–130 (2015)
63. D. Guha, D. Chakraborty, A new approach to fuzzy distance measure and similarity measure between two generalized fuzzy numbers. Appl. Soft Comput. **10**(1), 90–99 (2010)
64. E. Van Broekhoven, B. De Baets, Fast and accurate center of gravity defuzzification of fuzzy system outputs defined on trapezoidal fuzzy partitions. Fuzzy Sets Syst. **157**(7), 904–918 (2006)

65. T. Chen, Ubiquitous hotel recommendation using a fuzzy-weighted-average and back-propagation-network approach. Int. J. Intell. Syst. **32**, 316–341 (2017)
66. T. Chen, Ubiquitous multicriteria clinic recommendation system. J. Med. Syst. **40**(5), 113 (2016)
67. Y.C. Wang, T. Chen, Adapted techniques of explainable artificial intelligence for explaining genetic algorithms on the example of job scheduling. Expert Syst. Appl. 121369 (2023)
68. Y.C. Lin, Y.C. Wang, T.C.T. Chen, H.F. Lin, Evaluating the suitability of a smart technology application for fall detection using a fuzzy collaborative intelligence approach. Mathematics **7**(11), 1097 (2019)

Chapter 5
XAmI Applications to Telemedicine and Telecare

Abstract Telemedicine and telecare are another important application of ambient intelligence (AmI). This chapter first summarizes the applications of artificial intelligence (AI) in telemedicine and telecare. Since some of these AI applications are difficult to understand or communicate with patients, various explainable ambient intelligence (XAmI) techniques have been applied, such as shape-added explanation value (SHAP) analysis and locally interpretable model-agnostic explanation (LIME) to overcome such difficulties. Telemedicine services for type-II diabetes diagnosis are taken as an example to illustrate such applications. Several issues with existing XAmI applications in telemedicine and telecare are then discussed. It is worth noting that after SHAP analysis, some important attributes may be difficult to measure by patients themselves, which affects the utility of telemedicine or telecare applications.

Keywords Explainable artificial intelligence · Telemedicine · Telecare · Shapely additive explanation value · Locally interpretable model-agnostic explanations

5.1 Artificial Intelligence (AI) Applications in Telemedicine and Telecare

Telemedicine and telecare services have shown their effectiveness in mitigating the impact of the COVID-19 pandemic [1–4]. Telemedicine and telenursing services are a type of smart health technology dedicated to providing medical examinations (or tests) to patients in schools, companies, homes, and other places with the patient's consent [5–6]. These medical examinations are performed remotely by medical professionals through modern telecommunications means [7]. However, in order to accurately diagnose the disease a patient may have, specific sophisticated equipment is often required, which is only available in medical centers and used by professionals. This situation can lead to the following phenomena [5, 8]:

- There is a limit to the number of patients a physician can examine.
- Patients are experiencing increased wait times to get appointments [9–12].
- A certain number of tests are required before a diagnosis can be made.

© The Author(s), under exclusive license to Springer Nature Switzerland AG 2024
T.-C. T. Chen, *Explainable Ambient Intelligence (XAmI)*,
SpringerBriefs in Applied Sciences and Technology,
https://doi.org/10.1007/978-3-031-54935-9_5

To address these issues, **artificial intelligence (AI)** has been widely applied in telemedicine and telecare.

For example, Taleb-Ahmed et al. [5] established an online vision testing system in which the patient stood 5 m away from his/her computer screen and clicked the left or right button depending on whether he saw an open or closed C character. The answer was then transmitted back to the doctor's computer. Since the patient might be unsure of the characters he/she saw, visual acuity measurements were modeled as **fuzzy sets** to account for this uncertainty [13–16].

Fuzzy inference systems (FISs) [17–20] are another fuzzy logic application in telemedicine and telecare. In the telemedicine system developed by Nagayo et al. [21], biosensors and switches were attached to a patient to detect his/her body temperature, oxygen saturation, systemic arterial pressure, breathing pattern, pulse (heart rate), supplemental oxygen dependence, consciousness, and pain level. After the detection results were transmitted to the backend, a **Mamdani FIS** [22] was built to assess the patient's health risk to assist medical professionals in deciding appropriate clinical interventions.

Early diagnosis of epilepsy can help reduce the risk of death and eliminate post-traumatic difficulties. To this end, Kadu et al. [23] attached sensors to patients with epilepsy to collect medical data including air quality, body acceleration, breathing rate, heart rate, blood oxygen levels, and body temperature. These data were fed into a **machine learning (ML)** method [24], the gradient boosting decision tree (GBDT) algorithm, to predict patient health status.

Telemedicine systems that transmit medical signals such as electrocardiograms (ECG) and electroencephalograms (EEG) over long distances must compress these signals to efficiently utilize bandwidth. In Sriram [25], three **artificial neural networks (ANNs)** [26–27], namely single-layer perceptron (SLP), multi-layer perceptron (MLP), and Elman network (EN), were constructed to estimate the original medical signal from the received compressed signal. After comparison, SLP achieves the best performance by maximizing the correlation between the original medical signals and the reconstructed medical signals.

In telemedicine systems, in order to protect patient privacy, it is usually necessary to encrypt medical images transmitted through communication networks. This encryption needs to meet several criteria, including balance, high nonlinearity, low differential uniformity, and low autocorrelation, which leads to intractable multi-objective optimization problems. To help address this issue, Ahmad et al. [28] proposed a chaos-assisted non-dominated sorting **genetic algorithm (GA)**-II. In this way, multiple Pareto optimal solutions could be derived, which enhanced the flexibility of implementation.

A similar telemedicine system was built in Chiu and Chen [7], in which multiple 3D printing facilities collaborated for making dentures. The telemedicine system received orders from dental clinics and then distributed the dentures to be printed among 3D printing facilities to save time. Unlike that of Ahmad et al. [28], patient data transmitted through the telemedicine system are the 3D computer-aided design (CAD) files [29] of the dentals of patients. In addition, compared with existing systems for similar purposes, the telemedicine system still had two novel features.

The first was the consideration of the possibility of reprinting in formulating the plan to avoid replanning. The other was the cooperation with home delivery services that have gradually become popular during the COVID-19 pandemic to save transportation time. The new features were subject to considerable uncertainties. To account for the uncertainties, both printing time and transportation time were modeled using interval type-II trapezoidal fuzzy numbers. Subsequently, an interval type-II **fuzzy mixed integer-linear programming (FMILP)** model was formulated and optimized to plan the operations of the telemedicine system.

Chen et al. [30] established a telemedicine system for fabricating prosthetics. The 3D CAD file of a patient's prosthetic limb was transferred to the appropriate 3D printing facility [31]. To this end, the physician applied the **modified evolutionary fuzzy assessment (MEFA)** method on behalf of the patient to derive the fuzzy priorities of criteria. Subsequently, in order to eliminate the dependence between the criteria, **principal component analysis (PCA)** was applied. Finally, the dependency-removed **fuzzy technique for order preference via similarity to ideal solutions (FTOPSIS)** (Dr-FTOPSIS) was proposed to evaluate and compare the 3D printing facilities under consideration.

Figure 5.1 provides statistics on the popularity of AI technology applications in telemedicine and telecare. AI technologies most widely used in telemedicine and telecare include k-means, deep learning, and case-based reasoning.

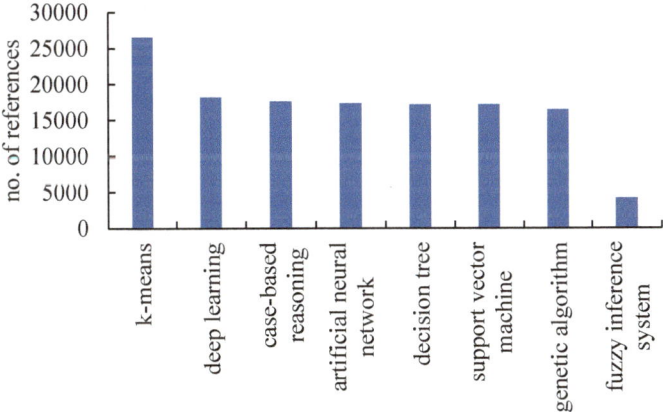

Fig. 5.1 Number of references about AI technology applications in telemedicine and telecare from 2013 to 2023 (Data source Google Scholar)

5.2   Effectiveness of AI Applications for Telemedicine and Telecare Services

All in all, AI has shown its effectiveness in supporting telemedicine or telecare services, as shown in the example below.

Example 5.1 (**AI Application in Diabetes Diagnosis**) The diabetes dataset from the National Institute of Diabetes and Digestive and Kidney Diseases (NIDDKD) [32] is used to demonstrate the calculation of SHAP values. The purpose of this dataset is to diagnostically predict whether a patient has diabetes based on certain diagnostic measurements. The dataset contains 768 instances selected from a large database (see Table 5.1) subject to several limitations. In particular, all patients were females of Pima Indian heritage who were at least 21 years old. In this example, the probability of patient j having type-II diabetes, a_j, is to be predicted based on the values of eight patient attributes, $x_{j1} \sim x_{j8}$ (see Table 5.2), using an ANN. If $a_j = 1$, patient j has type-II diabetes; otherwise, the patient does not have type-II diabetes. The ANN has three layers: the input layer, a single hidden layer (with up to sixteen nodes), and an output layer (see Fig. 5.2). The Levenberg–Marquardt (LM) algorithm [33] is applied to train the ANN using MATLAB. The maximum number of epochs is 20000. The target for RMSE is less than 0.25, or mean squared error (MSE) < 0.625:

$$\text{RMSE} = \sqrt{\frac{\sum_{j=1}^{n} (o_j - a_j)^2}{n}} \tag{5.1}$$

Data of the first 576 patients is used as the training data, while the remaining data is left for testing. The MATLAB code is shown in Fig. 5.3. The forecasting results are summarized in Fig. 5.4. The RMSE for test data is 0.43, which provides a **global explanation** of the AI application (i.e., the ANN) [34]. In addition, a **local explanation** for the diagnosis process and result of patient #749 is.

The probability that patient #749 has type-II diabetes predicted using the ANN is 0.658.

which is a **black-box explanation**.

Table 5.1   Type-II diabetes-related data of 768 patients [32]

j	x_{j1}	x_{j2}	x_{j3}	x_{j4}	x_{j5}	x_{j6}	x_{j7}	x_{j8}	a_j
1	6	148	72	35	0	33.6	0.627	50	1
2	1	85	66	29	0	26.6	0.351	31	0
3	8	183	64	0	0	23.3	0.672	32	1
...									
768	1	93	70	31	0	30.4	0.315	23	0

Table 5.2 Patient attributes

Attribute	Meaning
x_{j1}	Number of pregnancies
x_{j2}	Glucose level in blood
x_{j3}	Blood pressure measurement
x_{j4}	Thickness of skin
x_{j5}	Insulin level in blood
x_{j6}	Body mass index
x_{j7}	Diabetes percentage
x_{j8}	Age

Fig. 5.2 Architecture of the ANN

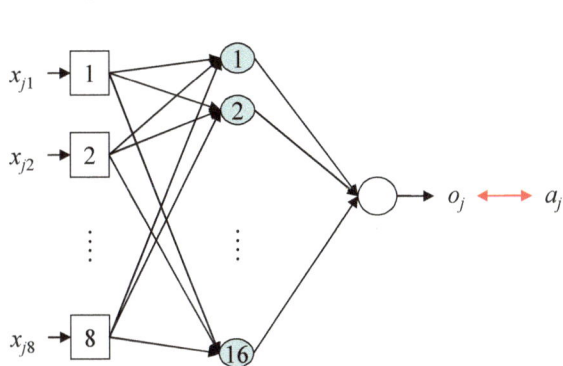

Patients with $o_j \geq 0.5$ are diagnosed as having type-II diabetes, while patients with $o_j < 0.5$ are diagnosed as not having type-II diabetes. The **confusion matrix**, another global XAmI tool, is constructed in Fig. 5.5. The classification performance can be evaluated in terms of the following measures

$$\text{Precision} = \frac{\text{true positive}}{\text{true positive} + \text{false positive}} \tag{5.2}$$

$$\text{Recall} = \frac{\text{true positive}}{\text{true positive} + \text{false negative}} \tag{5.3}$$

$$F1 = \frac{1}{\frac{\frac{1}{\text{precision}} + \frac{1}{\text{recall}}}{2}} \tag{5.4}$$

$$\text{Hamming loss} = \frac{\text{false positive} + \text{false negative}}{\text{all}} \tag{5.5}$$

```
% Colleated data
train_x=diabetesexample(1:576,1:8);
train_y=diabetesexample(1:576,9:9);
test_x=diabetesexample(577:768,1:8);
test_y=diabetesexample(577:768,9:9);
train_x=transpose(train_x);
train_y=transpose(train_y);
test_x=transpose(test_x);
test_y=transpose(test_y);

% ANN configuration
net1=feedforwardnet([16]);
net1.dividefcn='dividetrain'; % allocate all samples to the training data
net1.trainParam.lr=0.1;
net1.trainParam.epochs=20000;
net1.trainParam.goal=0.625;

% Training
net1=train(net1,train_x,train_y);

% Forecasting
train_o=net1(train_x);
test_o=net1(test_x);

% Accuracy evaluation
test_rmse=mean((test_y-test_o).^2)^0.5
```

Fig. 5.3 MATLAB code for implementing the ANN

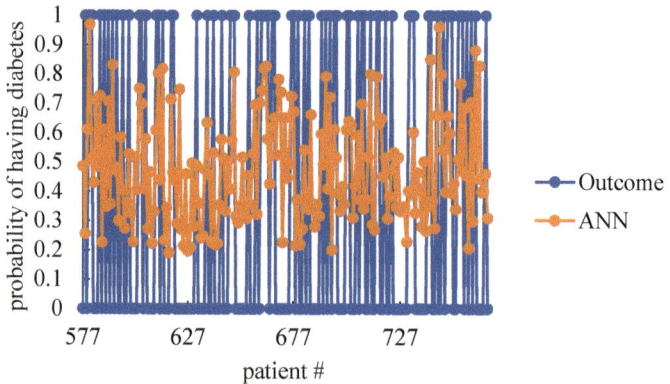

Fig. 5.4 Forecasting results

as precision = 66%; recall rate = 73%; F1 = 69%; Hamming loss = 0.234. All measures are the higher the better and also provide **global explanations** of the ANN.

The following discusses the situation when the diagnosis is performed through telemedicine services.

Fig. 5.5 Confusion matrix

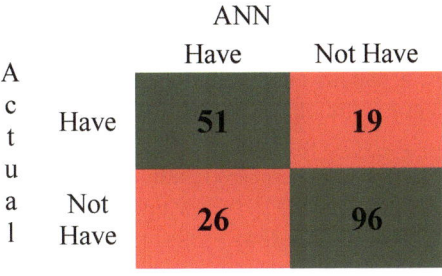

Example 5.2 (**Telemedicine as a Service**) In the previous example, when the diagnosis is performed through a telemedicine service, certain attributes are difficult to measure by patients themselves, such as x_{j4} (the thickness of skin) and x_{j7} (diabetes pedigree function result). In this case, a treatment is to replace the missing value of the attribute with its mean value. For example, if patient #749 uses the telemedicine service for a type-II diabetes diagnosis, while his skin thickness and diabetes pedigree function outcomes cannot be measured (or calculated). Therefore, the values of these two attributes are replaced by their average values of 20.54 and 0.472, respectively:

$$\{3, \ 187, \ 70, \ X, \ 200, \ 36.4, \ X, \ 36\}$$
$$\rightarrow \{3, \ 187, \ 70, \ 20.54, \ 200, \ 36.4, \ 0.472, \ 36\}$$

After predicting his probability of developing type-II diabetes using the ANN, the result is 0.657. In contrast, if the values of all attributes are known, the probability is 0.658. Obviously, the difference between the two diagnostic results is very small, showing the robustness of the ANN as an inference mechanism for the telemedicine service.

5.3 Explainable Ambient Intelligence (XAmI) Applications in Telemedicine and Telecare

The use of explainable ambient intelligence (XAmI) in telemedicine and telecare is apparently uncommon. Some examples are given below.

Lo Giudice et al. [35] constructed a convolutional neural network (CNN) to process the respiratory sounds (including normal respiratory cycles, crackles, wheezes, etc.) of patients transmitted through the communication network to diagnosis whether or not the patients had specific respiratory conditions. To explain the reasoning mechanism of the CNN, the **gradient-weighted class activation mapping (Grad-CAM)** technique was applied. The Grad-CAM technique was similar to a **heatmap** [36], which visualized the parts of a sonogram emphasized by the CNN in disease classification.

Wang et al. [36] constructed an ANN to diagnose whether a patient has type-II diabetes. The ANN runs on the server (or doctor) side and could be accessed by a patient using an app on his/her smartphone. Some inputs to the artificial neural network were measured on the patient side, while other inputs came from the patient's medical records on the server side. To facilitate communication of the diagnostic process and results to patients, Wang et al. approximated the ANN using **decision trees** [37], following the concept of **locally interpretable model-agnostic explanations (LIME)** [38].

Teleophthalmology is one of the mainstreams of telemedicine and telecare. Obayya et al. [39] established a teleophthalmology system for diabetic retinopathy grading and classification, in which a bidirectional gated recurrent convolutional unit (BGRCU) was constructed and optimized using the Archimedes optimization algorithm (AOA). A **confusion matrix** was used to illustrate the overall classification performance to provide a global explanation [40].

Qomariyah and Kazakov [41] built an AI-based telemedicine system for detecting COVID-19. Users used the application to submit medical data (including chest X-ray (CXR), lung computed tomography (CT) scan, and blood sample data). Then, the telemedicine system used three deep neural networks (DNNs) to predict a user's probability of contracting COVID-19 and responded to the user with the result through the same app. Qomariyah and Kazakov conducted a **Shapely additive explanation value (SHAP) analysis** and drew a **force plot** to determine and illustrate the importance levels of various attributes in COVID-19 diagnosis [42–43]. In addition, three XAmI technologies, **decision tree, random forest (RF)**, and **extreme gradient boosting (XGBoost)**, were applied to approximate the reasoning mechanisms of the deep neural networks to generate easy-to-communicate diagnosis rules [44–45].

Generally speaking, explanations in XAmI can be divided into the following categories: global explanations, local explanations, contrastive explanations, hypothetical explanations, exemplar-based explanations, and model-agnostic explanations. From a different perspective, He et al. [46] classified user requirements for XAmI in healthcare into seven categories: input, efficacy, if/how to be that/how to still be that, output, how (global), and why/why not. Telemedicine or telecare services may encounter problems gathering information, which can complicate the diagnostic process and reduce efficacy, making it difficult to interpret other items.

Despite the growing market for fertility services, infertility evaluation remains uncomfortable, expensive, inaccessible, and unclear for both clients and fertility service providers. Therefore, teleconsultation can be used to eliminate possible embarrassment. Marvin and Alarm [47] applied quantum lattice learning to build a lattice model that predicts fertility treatment outcomes. They then drew an association diagram to illustrate the rules used in the prediction process. A confusion matrix was also built to show the classification accuracy of the proposed methodology.

5.4 Popular XAmI Techniques for Telemedicine and Telecare

5.4.1 SHAP

In sum, SHAP analysis is definitely the most popular XAmI technique. The SHAP value can then be defined as the weighted average of the marginal contributions of all possible coalitions $|\mathbf{F}|!$ as [48]

$$\varphi_m(f) = \sum_{\{\mathbf{S} \subseteq \mathbf{F}\} \setminus \{m\}} \frac{|\mathbf{S}|!(|\mathbf{F}| - |\mathbf{S}| - 1)!}{|\mathbf{F}|!} \cdot [f(x_{\mathbf{S} \cup \{m\}}) - f(x_{\mathbf{S}})] \tag{5.6}$$

where $\varphi_m(f)$ is the weighted average Shapley value that feature m provides in the context of all coalitions that exclude feature m. $\mathbf{F}$ is the set of all features; $\mathbf{S}$ is a subset (i.e., coalition) of $\mathbf{F}$; $f(x_{\mathbf{S} \cup \{m\}})$ is the model prediction considering feature m, while $f(x_{\mathbf{S}})$ is the model prediction without considering feature m.

The Shapley value of a patient's attribute reflects the impact of this attribute on the patient's diagnosis result and is determined as follows:

Step 1. Consider the first attribute.
Step 2. Fix the value of the attribute, and randomize the values of the other attributes to generate random data.
Step 3. Apply the trained AI model to diagnose each randomly generated data.
Step 4. Calculate the average value of the diagnosis results:

$$\overline{o}_j(m) = \frac{\sum_{t=1}^{T} o_{jt}(m)}{T} \tag{5.7}$$

where $o_{jt}(m)$ is the diagnosis result of random data t by fixing attribute m of patient j.
Step 5. Subtract the average result from the diagnosis result of the patient, and divide the result by M, where M is the number of attributes:

$$\text{SHAP}_{jm} = o_j - \overline{o}_j(m) \tag{5.8}$$

where o_j is the diagnosis result of patient j. The result gives the Shapley value of attribute m for the patient.
Step 6. Consider the next attribute, and return to Step 2.

A SHAP analysis can be performed to make a local explanation [42, 49]. The average importance of an attribute for all jobs can be derived:

$$SHAP_m = \frac{1}{n} \sum_{j=1}^{n} SHAP_{jm} \qquad (5.9)$$

Example 5.3 (**SHAP Application in Diabetes Diagnosis**) In Example 5.1, the SHAP value of each patient attribute is derived and the results are summarized in Table 5.3. The required MATLAB code is provided in Fig. 5.6. A **force plot** can be plotted to summarize the results of the SHAP analysis (see Fig. 5.7). To accurately predict the chance of developing type-II diabetes, attributes with higher absolute SHAP values are more important. For example, for patient #1, $x_{j2} \sim x_{j4}$ are more important in predicting whether the patient has type-II diabetes. Another XAmI tool for comparing the SHAP values of different attributes is a **tornado plot**, as shown in Fig. 5.8.

Example 5.4 (**Telemedicine as a Service**) As noted in Example 5.2, x_{j4} (the thickness of skin) is difficult to measure by the patient herself. As a result,

- The patient may need to go to the hospital to measure the attribute for accurate diagnosis.
- The patient may focus on improving other attributes that are both important and self-measurable.

Table 5.3 SHAP values of patient attributes

j	$SHAP_{j1}$	$SHAP_{j2}$	$SHAP_{j3}$	$SHAP_{j4}$	$SHAP_{j5}$	$SHAP_{j6}$	$SHAP_{j7}$	$SHAP_{j8}$
1	− 0.006	− 0.027	− 0.023	− 0.014	− 0.006	− 0.005	− 0.008	− 0.006
2	− 0.026	− 0.057	− 0.057	− 0.058	− 0.032	− 0.065	− 0.079	− 0.093
3	− 0.002	0.029	0.017	0.006	0.010	0.013	0.010	− 0.023
...								
576	− 0.021	− 0.037	− 0.043	− 0.036	− 0.003	0.048	0.059	− 0.007

```
% Derive SHAP values
SHAPvalues=zeros(576,8);
eval_x=zeros(8,1);
for i=1:576
    eval_x=train_x(1:8,i);
    for j=1:8
    eval_sum=0;
        for k=1:100
            eval_x(j,1)=min(train_x(j,:))+rand*(max(train_x(j,:))-min(train_x(j,:)));
            eval_o=net1(eval_x);
            eval_sum=eval_sum+eval_o;
        end
        SHAPvalues(i,j)=(train_o(1,i)-eval_sum/100)/8;
    end
end
```

Fig. 5.6 MATLAB code for deriving the SHAP values of patient attributes

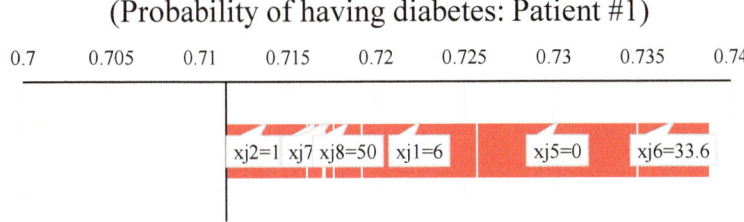

Fig. 5.7 Force plot

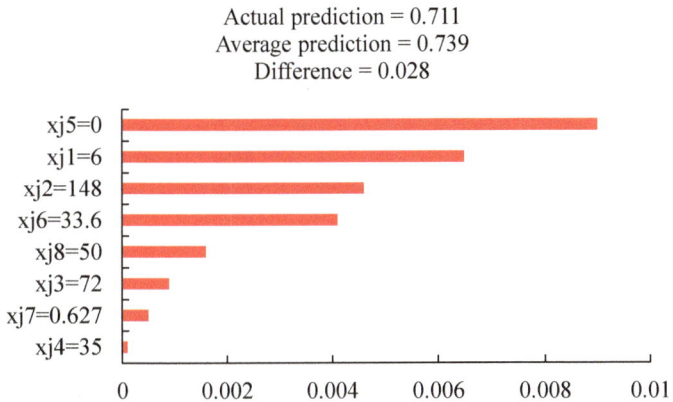

Fig. 5.8 Tornado plot

There are other methods for evaluating the impact, contribution, or importance of each patient attribute on the diagnosis outcome, such as [34].

- correlation analysis, back elimination of regression analysis, contingency table analysis, etc.,
- partial derivation,
- odd ratio,
- out-of-bag (OOB) predictor importance,
- recursive feature elimination (RFE), and
- permutation feature importance (PFI).

5.4.2   LIME with Decision Tree (DT) Application

LIME is to approximate a globally complex AI model with multiple locally simpler ones [38, 50]. LIME minimizes the following objective function:

$$\text{Min}\, \xi(x) = \arg\min_{g \in G} L(f, g, \pi_x) + \Omega(g) \qquad (5.10)$$

where f and g indicate the original and interpretation models, respectively. π_x measures the proximity from all approximate outcomes to the original outputs. argmin() returns the g value that minimizes $L()$. $\Omega()$ is a measure of model complexity.

The steps of LIME are as follows:

- conduct pre-model data analysis,
- train the AI model,
- generate synthetic data,
- apply the trained AI model to synthetic data,
- approximate the AI application (i.e., fit synthetic data),
- evaluate the explanation performance.

Both ANNs and decision trees (DTs) can be applied individually to predict the probability of a patient having diabetes [21]. However, ANNs, especially with deep learning, generally perform better than DTs [48, 51]. Nevertheless, DTs are simple and easy to understand and communicate.

The concept of LIME can be followed to construct a DT to approximate the ANN for diabetes diagnosis, rather than just applying the two methods individually. In this way, the prediction mechanism of the ANN in each local area of the solution space can be fitted using the simple decision rules of the DT, avoiding the possible overfitting problem of the ANN, thereby reducing misclassification and enhancing diagnosis accuracy. Traditionally, the outcome of a decision rule is given by the ANN outputs of all patients to whom the decision rule applies:

$$\hat{o}_k(b) = \frac{\sum_{j \in \Omega(b, k)} o_j}{\sum_{j \in \Omega(b, k)} 1} \qquad (5.11)$$

$\Omega(b, k)$ is the set of patients to whom the k-th decision rule of decision tree b applies.

Example 5.5 (**Synthetic Data Generation**) Before using a DT to approximate the ANN, it is usually necessary to generate synthetic data to avoid the effects of extreme cases, data imbalance, and missing values [52]. In this case, synthetic data is generated through randomization. The required MATLAB code is shown in Fig. 5.9.

Example 5.6 (**LIME Application in Diabetes Diagnosis**) A DT is constructed to approximate the ANN for diabetes diagnosis in Example 5.1 based on the synthetic data generated in Example 5.5. The required MATLAB code is shown in Fig. 5.10. The constructed DT is illustrated in Fig. 5.11, with decision rules summarized in

```
% Randomization
synthetic_x=zeros(1000,8);
for i=1:1000
    for j=1:8
        synthetic_x(i,j)=rand()*(max(train_x(:,j))-min(train_x(:,j)))+min(train_x(:,j));
    end
end
synthetic_o=net1(transpose(synthetic_x));
```

Fig. 5.9 MATLAB code for generating synthetic data

```
% Approximate the ANN with a DT
DT_x=synthetic_x;
DT_y=transpose(synthetic_o);
DT1=fitrtree(DT_x,DT_y);
view(DT1,'Mode','text');
view(DT1,'Mode','graph');
synthetic_oh=predict(DT1,DT_x);
```

Fig. 5.10 MATLAB code for approximating the ANN with a DT

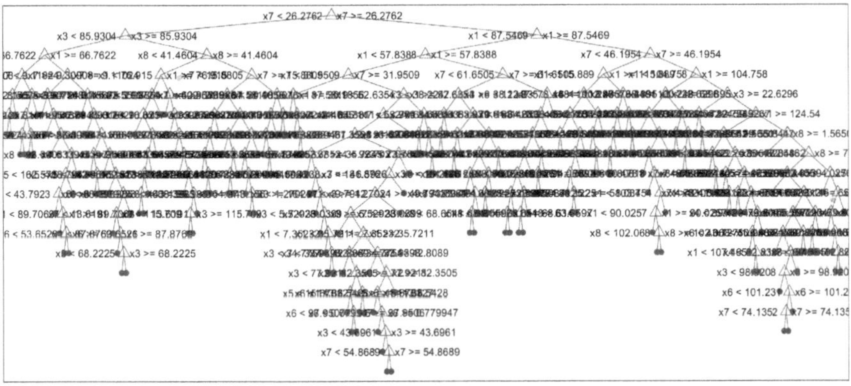

Fig. 5.11 DT constructed for approximating the ANN

Fig. 5.12. There are 170 rules in this case. For each patient, only one decision rule is applicable. For example, the decision rule applicable for patient #1 and can be communicated with the patient is:

$$\text{If } x_7 < 12.91 \text{ and } x_8 < 57.95 \text{ and } x_2 \geq 56.82 \text{ Then } \hat{o}_j = 0.7078.$$

while $o_j = 0.7115$. After removing technical terms,

If your diabetes percentage is higher than 12.91, you are over 57.95 years old, and your blood sugar level is above 56.82, then your chance of developing diabetes is 0.7078.

1	if x7<26.0372 then node 2 elseif x7>=26.0372 then node 3 else 0.374293
2	if x1<55.7957 then node 4 elseif x1>=55.7957 then node 5 else 0.617785
3	if x1<71.9244 then node 6 elseif x1>=71.9244 then node 7 else 0.279131
4	if x7<12.9117 then node 8 elseif x7>=12.9117 then node 9 else 0.465506
5	if x3<141.448 then node 10 elseif x3>=141.448 then node 11 else 0.699333
6	if x1<54.8565 then node 12 elseif x1>=54.8565 then node 13 else 0.127216
7	if x7<47.4844 then node 14 elseif x7>=47.4844 then node 15 else 0.426468
8	if x8<57.9471 then node 16 elseif x8>=57.9471 then node 17 else 0.700363
9	if x3<90.2558 then node 18 elseif x3>=90.2558 then node 19 else 0.28189
10	if x1<80.5077 then node 20 elseif x1>=80.5077 then node 21 else 0.658279
...	
337	fit = 0.104827
338	fit = 0.460244
339	fit = 0.450141

Fig. 5.12   Decision rules of the DT

Example 5.7 (**Telemedicine as a Service**) In Example 5.2, when patient #749 uses the diabetes diagnosis telemedicine service, x_{j4} (the thickness of skin) and x_{j7} (diabetes pedigree function result) are difficult to measure by herself. Therefore, a decision rule containing the two attributes cannot be used to explain the prediction process and result using the ANN. Instead, a DT containing the other attributes needs to be fitted. The required MATLAB code is shown in Fig. 5.13. The decision rules are summarized in Fig. 5.14. There are 115 rules in this case.

```
% Remove x4 and x7
DT_x=transpose(train_x([1:3,5:6,8],:));
DT_y=transpose(train_o);
DT1=fitrtree(DT_x,DT_y);
view(DT1,'Mode','text');
view(DT1,'Mode','graph');
synthetic_oh=predict(DT1,DT_x);
```

Fig. 5.13   MATLAB code

1	if x1<6.5 then node 2 elseif x1>=6.5 then node 3 else 0.463419
2	if x2<131.5 then node 4 elseif x2>=131.5 then node 5 else 0.400221
3	if x2<133.5 then node 6 elseif x2>=133.5 then node 7 else 0.691437
4	if x8<27.5 then node 8 elseif x8>=27.5 then node 9 else 0.344147
5	if x8<24.5 then node 10 elseif x8>=24.5 then node 11 else 0.540188
6	if x1<9.5 then node 12 elseif x1>=9.5 then node 13 else 0.60515
7	if x5<14.5 then node 14 elseif x5>=14.5 then node 15 else 0.804889
8	if x6<28.15 then node 16 elseif x6>=28.15 then node 17 else 0.297118
9	if x8<53 then node 18 elseif x8>=53 then node 19 else 0.416355
10	if x6<31.3 then node 20 elseif x6>=31.3 then node 21 else 0.428682
...	
227	if x5<129.5 then node 228 elseif x5>=129.5 then node 229 else 0.388901
228	fit = 0.415801
229	fit = 0.385912

Fig. 5.14   Decision rules that do not contain x_{j4} and x_{j7}

From Example 5.6, it is worth noting that the number of decision rules increases after removing two attributes since the ANN needs to be explained with fewer attributes. In other words, when diabetes diagnosis is provided as a telemedicine service, the local explanations provided to patients will be more diverse.

5.4.3 LIME with Random Forest (RF) Application

However, like other telemedicine and telecare services, using ANN for diabetes diagnosis is a big data problem, and a single DT may not be accurate enough to approximate an ANN. To solve this problem, a RF composed of several DTs can be constructed. Each decision tree considers a random subset of attributes (i.e., feature bagging) and is trained with examples randomly selected from the data with replacement (i.e., bootstrapping) [53–54]. In each DT, there is a decision rule that applies to a certain patient. The outcomes of the decision rules in all DTs applicable to the patient are averaged to generate a representative forecast.

Example 5.8 (**LIME Application with RF**) A RF composed of 10 DTs is constructed instead to approximate the ANN for diabetes diagnosis in Example 5.1 based on the synthetic data generated in Example 5.5. The required MATLAB code is shown in Fig. 5.15. The constructed RF is illustrated in Fig. 5.16, with decision rules summarized in Fig. 5.17.

Decision rules extracted using DT or RF may not be reasonable and need to be verified by a physician or domain expert [1, 9, 55]. A mobile application can also be designed to assist patients in transmitting self-measured data, and after the doctor approves, the diagnosis process and result will be reported to the patient (see Fig. 5.18).

Shen et al. [56] presented the prediction in words (i.e., textual description), and compared the two probabilities (the probabilities of having and not having diabetes) in a donut chart, as illustrated in Fig. 5.19.

Figure 5.20 summarizes popular AI and XAmI approaches in telemedicine and telecare. A closed loop exists, suggesting that user experience based on appropriate interpretations can be fed back to improve AI applications in the field [57–58].

```
% Approximate the ANN with a RF
RF1=TreeBagger(10,synthetic_x,transpose(synthetic_o),Method="regression",OOBPrediction="on");
synthetic_oh=predict(RF1,synthetic_x);

% Show the first DT
view(RF1.Trees{1},'Mode','graph');
view(RF1.Trees{1},'Mode','text');
```

Fig. 5.15 MATLAB code for approximating the ANN with a RF

(1st DT)

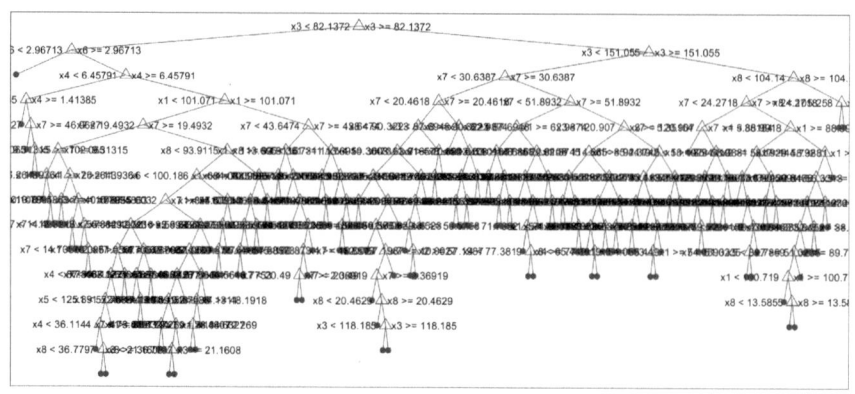

(2nd DT)

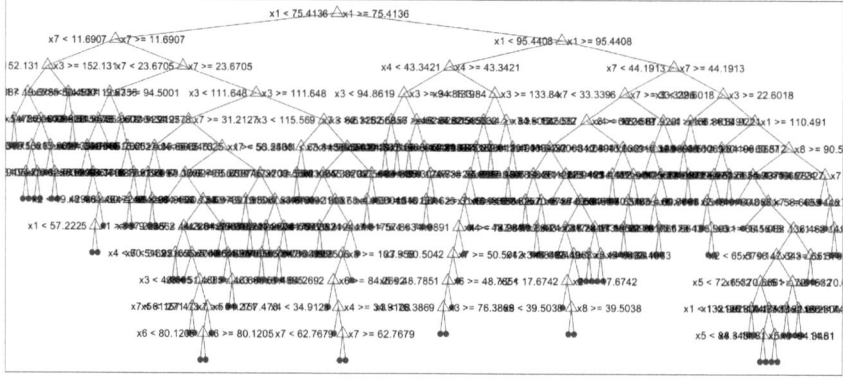

•••

(10th DT)

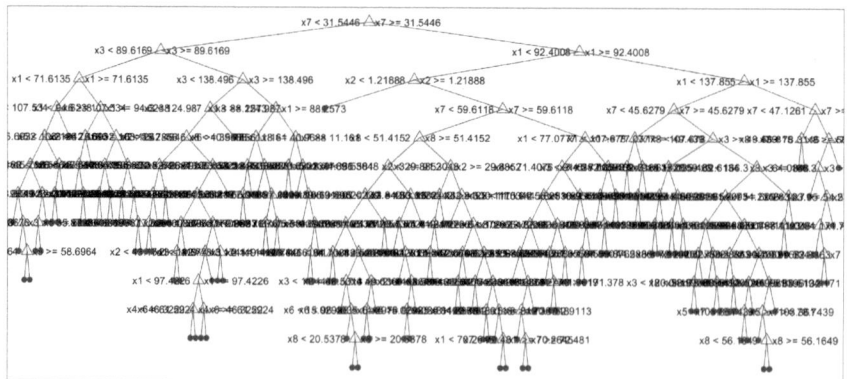

Fig. 5.16 RF constructed for approximating the ANN

(1st DT)
   1   if x8<81.9959 then node 2 elseif x8>=81.9959 then node 3 else 0.36349
   2   if x1<69.189 then node 4 elseif x1>=69.189 then node 5 else 0.336706
   3   if x7<51.2369 then node 6 elseif x7>=51.2369 then node 7 else 0.435905
...
289   fit = 0.382873
290   fit = 0.109344
291   fit = 0.0970812

(2nd DT)
   1   if x7<16.639 then node 2 elseif x7>=16.639 then node 3 else 0.381777
   2   if x1<61.2719 then node 4 elseif x1>=61.2719 then node 5 else 0.704218
   3   if x8<82.5173 then node 6 elseif x8>=82.5173 then node 7 else 0.306142
...
283   fit = 0.0972942
284   fit = 0.0961098
285   fit = 0.102457

...

(10th DT)
   1   if x7<26.0372 then node 2 elseif x7>=26.0372 then node 3 else 0.366277
   2   if x8<52.0769 then node 4 elseif x8>=52.0769 then node 5 else 0.617689
   3   if x3<27.9001 then node 6 elseif x3>=27.9001 then node 7 else 0.266063
...
273   fit = 0.388946
274   fit = 0.46367
275   fit = 0.428336

Fig. 5.17 Decision rules of the RF

5.5 Applicability Assessment of Telemedicine and Telecare Services Based on XAmI

When diagnosis is made through telemedicine services, certain attributes are difficult to accurately measure by the patients themselves. For example, in remote diabetes diagnosis services, it is difficult for patients to accurately measure skin thickness and diabetes spectrum function results by themselves. Therefore, the following XAmI-based approach can be applied to evaluate the applicability of telemedicine or telecare services:

- If according to the attribute impact assessment results, all the more influential attributes can be accurately measured by patients themselves, or are already in the medical records and do not need to be updated, then the applicability of this telemedicine or telecare service is high.

Fig. 5.18 User (patient)
interface of XAmI-based
telemedicine and telecare
system

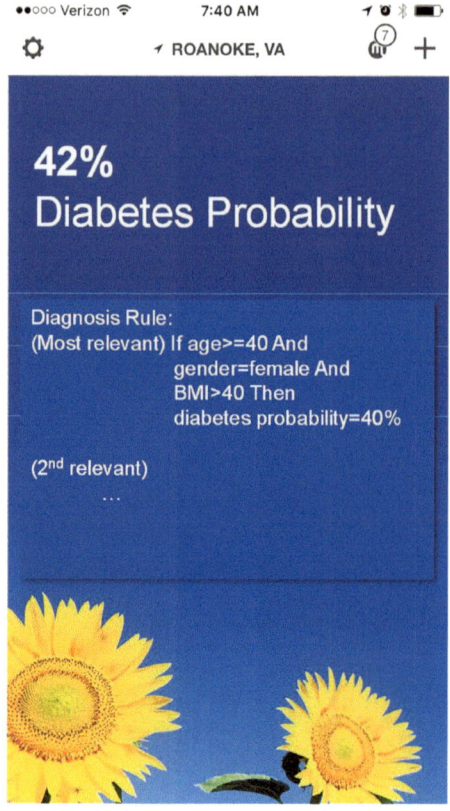

- This approach must meet other conditions, such as doctor availability, patient demand, the accuracy of the diagnosis mechanism, and government subsidies.

For diagnosis mechanisms built using different AI technologies, the more influential patient attributes may be different. In addition, the more influential patient attributes selected by different assessment methods may also be different. This is why various AI technologies and assessment methods need to be compared because they will affect the applicability assessment result of a telemedicine or telecare service (see Fig. 5.21).

Fig. 5.19 Comparing the
two probabilities in a donut
chart

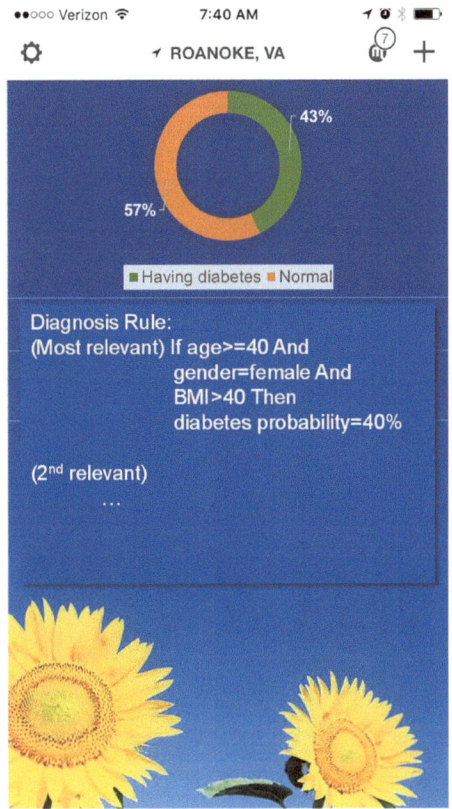

5.6   Issues with Existing XAmI Applications in Telemedicine and Telecare

Existing XAmI applications in telemedicine and telecare have the following problems:

- Telemedicine or telecare is a process involving big data [59–62]. There may be many patient attributes. Therefore, the importance of patient attributes may be diluted, making focusing on more critical patient attributes a challenging task [63–64].
- Most XAmI applications performed a SHAP analysis to identify the most critical attributes that were not properly utilized to increase the effectiveness of the AI technologies employed in the telemedicine or telecare systems [65–66].
- After the SHAP analysis, some important attributes may be difficult to measure by patients themselves, which affects the usefulness of telemedicine or healthcare applications.

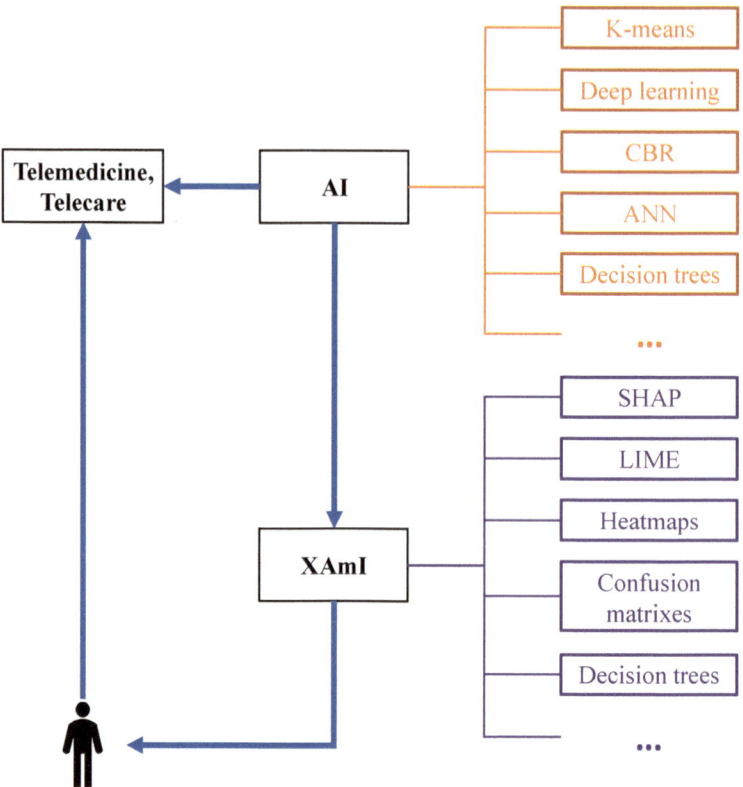

Fig. 5.20 Popular AI and XAmI approaches in telemedicine and telecare

- The potential of new telemedicine or telecare applications can be assessed in this way. The sustainability of existing telemedicine or telecare applications can also be examined [67–70].
- A single decision rule is not sufficient to explain the diagnostic mechanisms in telemedicine or telecare systems. However, multiple decision rules can lead to confusion for patients, who do not know which rule is most relevant [71–72].
- Another problem is that if there are many patients who need to use a telemedicine or telecare service, then how to sequence and schedule them is a challenging task [73–75] because the number of doctors is much less than the number of patients. However, sorting and scheduling are less discussed topics in XAmI applications, resulting in few successful cases for reference [76–81].

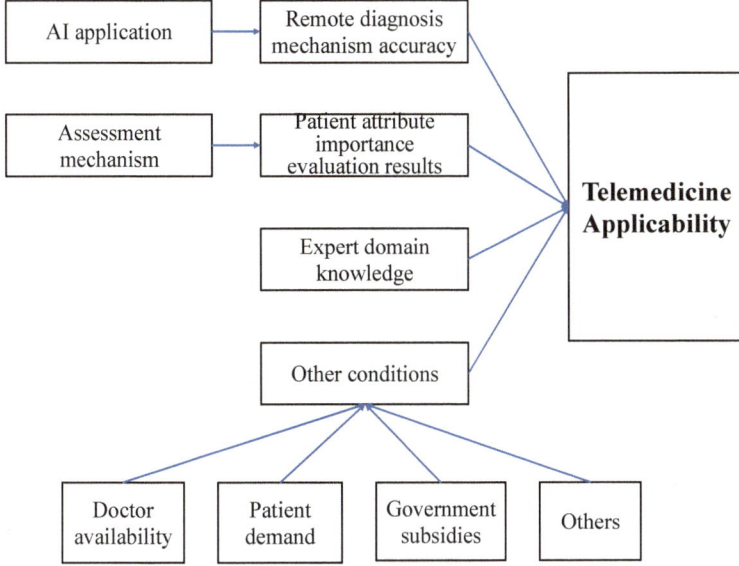

Fig. 5.21 XAmI-based applicability assessment mechanism for telemedicine or telecare services

References

1. T. Chen, C.W. Lin, Smart and automation technologies for ensuring the long-term operation of a factory amid the COVID-19 pandemic: an evolving fuzzy assessment approach. Int. J. Adv. Manuf. Technol. **111**, 3545–3558 (2020)
2. G. Battineni, G. Pallotta, G. Nittari, F. Amenta, Telemedicine framework to mitigate the impact of the COVID-19 pandemic. J. Taibah Univ. Med. Sci. **16**(2), 300 (2021)
3. H.C. Wu, Y.C. Wang, T.C.T. Chen, Assessing and comparing COVID-19 intervention strategies using a varying partial consensus fuzzy collaborative intelligence approach. Mathematics **8**(10), 1725 (2020)
4. T.C.T. Chen, in *Sustainable Smart Healthcare: Lessons Learned from the COVID-19 Pandemic.* Smart Technology Applications in Healthcare Before, During, and After the COVID-19 Pandemic (2023), pp. 19–37
5. A. Taleb-Ahmed, A. Bigand, V. Lethuc, P.M. Allioux, Visual acuity of vision tested by fuzzy logic: an application in ophthalmology as a step towards a telemedicine project. Inf. Fusion **5**(3), 217–230 (2004)
6. T.C.T. Chen, in *Sustainable Smart Healthcare: Lessons Learned from the COVID-19 Pandemic.* Smart Healthcare (2023), pp. 1–18
7. M.C. Chiu, T.C.T. Chen, A ubiquitous healthcare system of 3D printing facilities for making dentures: application of type-II fuzzy logic. Digital Health **8**, 20552076221092540 (2022)
8. T.C.T. Chen, in *Sustainable Smart Healthcare: Lessons Learned from the COVID-19 Pandemic.* Sustainable Smart Healthcare Applications: Lessons Learned from the COVID-19 Pandemic (2023), pp. 65–92
9. Y.C. Wang, T.C.T. Chen, A partial-consensus posterior-aggregation FAHP method—supplier selection problem as an example. Mathematics **7**(2), 179 (2019)
10. T. Chen, Y.C. Wang, H.C. Wu, Analyzing the impact of vaccine availability on alternative supplier selection amid the COVID-19 pandemic: a cFGM-FTOPSIS-FWI approach. Healthcare **9**(1), 71 (2021)

11. U. Naiker, G. FitzGerald, J.M. Dulhunty, M. Rosemann, Time to wait: a systematic review of strategies that affect out-patient waiting times. Aust. Health Rev. **42**(3), 286–293 (2017)

12. T.C.T. Chen, in *Production Planning and Control in Semiconductor Manufacturing: Big Data Analytics and Industry 4.0 Applications*. Job Sequencing and Scheduling (2023), pp. 77–90

13. G. Arji, H. Ahmadi, M. Nilashi, T.A. Rashid, O.H. Ahmed, N. Aljojo, A. Zainol, Fuzzy logic approach for infectious disease diagnosis: a methodical evaluation, literature and classification. Biocybern. Biomed. Eng. **39**(4), 937–955 (2019)

14. T. Chen, Y.C. Wang, M.C. Chiu, A type-II fuzzy collaborative forecasting approach for productivity forecasting under an uncertainty environment. J. Ambient. Intell. Humaniz. Comput. **12**, 2751–2763 (2021)

15. T. Djatna, M.K.D. Hardhienata, A.F.N. Masruriyah, An intuitionistic fuzzy diagnosis analytics for stroke disease. J. Big Data **5**, 1–14 (2018)

16. T. Chen, An innovative fuzzy and artificial neural network approach for forecasting yield under an uncertain learning environment. J. Ambient. Intell. Humaniz. Comput. **9**, 1013–1025 (2018)

17. S. Thukral, J.S. Bal, Medical applications on fuzzy logic inference system: a review. Int. J. Adv. Netw. Appl. **10**(4), 3944–3950 (2019)

18. T.C.T. Chen, Y.C. Wang, M.C. Chiu, An efficient approximating alpha-cut operations approach for deriving fuzzy priorities in fuzzy multi-criterion decision-making. Appl. Soft Comput. **139**, 110238 (2023)

19. I.B. de Medeiros, M.A.S. Machado, W.J. Damasceno, A.M. Caldeira, R.C. dos Santos, J.B. da Silva Filho, A fuzzy inference system to support medical diagnosis in real time. Proc. Comput. Sci. **122**, 167–173 (2017)

20. T.C.T. Chen, K. Honda, in *Fuzzy Collaborative Forecasting and Clustering: Methodology, System Architecture, and Applications*. Introduction to Fuzzy Collaborative Forecasting Systems (2020), pp. 1–8

21. A.M. Nagayo, M.Z.K. Al Ajmi, N.R.K. Guduri, F.S.H. AlBuradai, in *Proceedings of Third International Conference on Advances in Computer Engineering and Communication Systems*. IoT-Based Telemedicine Health Monitoring System with a Fuzzy Inference-Based Medical Decision Support Module for Clinical Risk Evaluation (2023), pp. 313–336

22. T.C.T. Chen, in *Sustainable Smart Healthcare: Lessons Learned from the COVID-19 Pandemic*. Enhancing the Sustainability of Smart Healthcare Applications with XAI (2023), pp. 93–110

23. A. Kadu, M. Singh, K. Ogudo, A novel scheme for classification of epilepsy using machine learning and a fuzzy inference system based on wearable-sensor health parameters. Sustainability **14**(22), 15079 (2022)

24. M.C. Chiu, T.C.T. Chen, K.W. Hsu, Modeling an uncertain productivity learning process using an interval fuzzy methodology. Mathematics **8**(6), 998 (2020)

25. N. Sriraam, Quality-on-demand compression of EEG signals for telemedicine applications using neural network predictors. Int. J. Telemed. Appl. **2011**, 860549 (2011)

26. Y.C. Lin, T. Chen, A ubiquitous clinic recommendation system using the modified mixed-binary nonlinear programming-feedforward neural network approach. J. Theor. Appl. Electron. Commer. Res. **16**(7), 3282–3298 (2021)

27. T. Chen, Y.C. Wang, A modified random forest incremental interpretation method for explaining artificial and deep neural networks in cycle time prediction. Decis. Anal. J. **7**, 100226 (2023)

28. M. Ahmad, R. Alkanhel, W. El-Shafai, A.D. Algarni, F.E. Abd El-Samie, N.F. Soliman, Multi-objective evolution of strong s-boxes using non-dominated sorting genetic algorithm-ii and chaos for secure telemedicine. IEEE Access **10**, 112757–112775 (2022)

29. Y.C. Wang, T. Chen, New XAI tools for selecting suitable 3D printing facilities in ubiquitous manufacturing. Compl. Intell. Syst. **9**, 6813–6829 (2023)

30. T.C.T. Chen, C.W. Lin, M.C. Chiu, Optimizing 3D printing facility selection for ubiquitous manufacturing using an evolving fuzzy big data analytics approach. Int. J. Adv. Manuf. Technol. **127**, 4111–4121 (2023)

31. Y.C. Wang, T. Chen, Y.C. Lin, 3D printer selection for aircraft component manufacturing using a nonlinear FGM and dependency-considered fuzzy VIKOR approach. Aerospace **10**(7), 591 (2023)

32. A.D. Khare, Diabetes dataset (2022). https://www.kaggle.com/datasets/akshaydattatraykhare/diabetes-dataset?resource=download
33. J. Nocedal, S. Wright, *Numerical Optimization* (Springer Science & Business Media, 2006)
34. T.C.T. Chen, in *Explainable Artificial Intelligence (XAI) in Manufacturing: Methodology, Tools, and Applications*. Applications of XAI for Forecasting in the Manufacturing Domain (2023), pp. 13–50
35. M. Lo Giudice, N. Mammone, C. Ieracitano, U. Aguglia, D. Mandic, F.C. Morabito, in *International Conference on Applied Intelligence and Informatics*. Explainable Deep Learning Classification of Respiratory Sound for Telemedicine Applications (2022), pp. 391–403
36. Y.C. Wang, T.C.T. Chen, M.C. Chiu, A systematic approach to enhance the explainability of artificial intelligence in healthcare with application to diagnosis of diabetes. Healthcare Anal. **3**, 100183 (2023)
37. T.C.T. Chen, in *Explainable Artificial Intelligence (XAI) in Manufacturing: Methodology, Tools, and Applications*. Applications of XAI for Decision Making in the Manufacturing Domain (2023), pp. 51–81
38. M.R. Zafar, N. Khan, Deterministic local interpretable model-agnostic explanations for stable explainability. Mach. Learn. Knowl. Extract. **3**(3), 525–541 (2021)
39. M. Obayya, N. Nemri, M.K. Nour, M. Al Duhayyim, H. Mohsen, M. Rizwanullah, et al., Explainable artificial intelligence enabled teleophthalmology for diabetic retinopathy grading and classification. Appl. Sci. **12**(17), 8749 (2022)
40. Y.C. Wang, T.C.T. Chen, M.C. Chiu, An improved explainable artificial intelligence tool in healthcare for hospital recommendation. Healthcare Anal. **3**, 100147 (2023)
41. N.N. Qomariyah, D.L. Kazakov, *Smart AI-Based Telemedicine System for Covid-19* (Cv Syntax Computama, 2021)
42. K. Debjit, M.S. Islam, M.A. Rahman, F.T. Pinki, R.D. Nath, S. Al-Ahmadi, et al., An improved machine-learning approach for COVID-19 prediction using Harris Hawks optimization and feature analysis using SHAP. Diagnostics **12**(5), 1023 (2022)
43. H.C. Wu, Y.C. Lin, T.C.T. Chen, Leisure agricultural park selection for traveler groups amid the COVID-19 pandemic. Agriculture **12**(1), 111 (2022)
44. J. Lötsch, D. Kringel, A. Ultsch, Explainable artificial intelligence (XAI) in biomedicine: making AI decisions trustworthy for physicians and patients. BioMed Inf. **2**(1), 1–17 (2021)
45. Y.C. Lin, T.C.T. Chen, Type-II fuzzy approach with explainable artificial intelligence for nature-based leisure travel destination selection amid the COVID-19 pandemic. Digital Health **8**, 20552076221106320 (2022)
46. X. He, Y. Hong, X. Zheng, Y. Zhang, What are the users' needs? Design of a user-centered explainable artificial intelligence diagnostic system. Int. J. Human Comput. Interact. **39**(7), 1519–1542 (2023)
47. G. Marvin, M.G.R. Alarm, in *IEEE International Conference on Biomedical Engineering, Computer and Information Technology for Health*. An Explainable Lattice Based Fertility Treatment Outcome Prediction Model for Telefertility (2021), pp. 64–68
48. L.P. Joseph, E.A. Joseph, R. Prasad, Explainable diabetes classification using hybrid Bayesian-optimized TabNet architecture. Comput. Biol. Med. **151**, 106178 (2022)
49. T.C.T. Chen, in *Explainable Artificial Intelligence (XAI) in Manufacturing: Methodology, Tools, and Applications*. Explainable Artificial Intelligence (XAI) in Manufacturing (2023), pp. 1–11
50. N.B. Kumarakulasinghe, T. Blomberg, J. Liu, A.S. Leao, P. Papapetrou, in *IEEE 33rd International Symposium on Computer-Based Medical Systems*. Evaluating Local Interpretable Model-Agnostic Explanations on Clinical Machine Learning Classification Models (2020), pp. 7–12
51. Y.C. Wang, T.C.T. Chen, H.C. Wu, A novel auto-weighting deep-learning fuzzy collaborative intelligence approach. Decis. Anal. J. **6**, 100186 (2023)
52. T.C.T. Chen, in *Production Planning and Control in Semiconductor Manufacturing: Big Data Analytics and Industry 4.0 Applications*. Industry 4.0 for Semiconductor Manufacturing (2022), pp. 21–40

53. V. Rodriguez-Galiano, M. Sanchez-Castillo, M. Chica-Olmo, M.J.O.G.R. Chica-Rivas, Machine learning predictive models for mineral prospectivity: an evaluation of neural networks, random forest, regression trees and support vector machines. Ore Geol. Rev. **71**, 804–818 (2015)
54. J. Brownlee, How to avoid overfitting in deep learning neural networks (2019). https://machin elearningmastery.com/introduction-to-regularization-to-reduce-overfitting-and-improve-gen eralization-error/
55. T. Chen, Y.C. Lin, M.C. Chiu, Approximating alpha-cut operations approach for effective and efficient fuzzy analytic hierarchy process analysis. Appl. Soft Comput. **85**, 105855 (2019)
56. J. Shen, J. Chen, Z. Zheng, J. Zheng, Z. Liu, J. Song, S.Y. Wong, X. Wang, M. Huang, P.-H. Fang, B. Jiang, W. Tsang, Z. He, T. Liu, B. Akinwunmi, C.C. Wang, C.J.P. Zhang, J. Huang, W.K. Ming, An innovative artificial intelligence–based app for the diagnosis of gestational diabetes mellitus (gdm-ai): development study. J. Med. Internet Res. **22**(9), e21573 (2020)
57. W.H.A. Ryu, M.G. Kerolus, V.C. Traynelis, Clinicians' user experience of telemedicine in neurosurgery during COVID-19. World Neurosurg. **146**, e359–e367 (2021)
58. T.C.T. Chen, T.C. Chang, Y.C. Wang, Improving people' health by burning low-pollution coal to improve air quality for thermal power generation. Digital Health **9**, 20552076231185280 (2023)
59. R.D. Kindle, O. Badawi, L.A. Celi, S. Sturland, Intensive care unit telemedicine in the era of big data, artificial intelligence, and computer clinical decision support systems. Crit. Care Clin. **35**(3), 483–495 (2019)
60. T.C.T. Chen, in *Production Planning and Control in Semiconductor Manufacturing: Big Data Analytics and Industry 4.0 Applications.* Big Data Analytics for Semiconductor Manufacturing (2022), pp. 1–19
61. J.B. Awotunde, A.E. Adeniyi, R.O. Ogundokun, G.J. Ajamu, P.O. Adebayo, in *Enhanced Telemedicine and E-health: Advanced IoT Enabled Soft Computing Framework.* MIoT-Based Big Data Analytics Architecture, Opportunities and Challenges for Enhanced Telemedicine Systems (2021), pp. 199–220
62. T. Chen, Y.C. Wang, Hybrid big data analytics and Industry 4.0 approach to projecting cycle time ranges. Int. J. Adv. Manuf. Technol. **120**(1–2), 279–295 (2022)
63. J. Driessen, A. Bonhomme, W. Chang, D.A. Nace, D. Kavalieratos, S. Perera, S.M. Handler, Nursing home provider perceptions of telemedicine for reducing potentially avoidable hospitalizations. J. Am. Med. Dir. Assoc. **17**(6), 519–524 (2016)
64. T.C.T. Chen, Y.C. Wang, in *Artificial Intelligence and Lean Manufacturing.* Basics in Lean Management (2022), pp. 1–12
65. K.M. Zobair, L. Sanzogni, L. Houghton, M.Z. Islam, Forecasting care seekers satisfaction with telemedicine using machine learning and structural equation modeling. PLoS ONE **16**(9), e0257300 (2021)
66. K. Prabhakaran, G. Lombardo, R. Latifi, Telemedicine for trauma and emergency management: an overview. Curr. Trauma Rep. **2**, 115–123 (2016)
67. E.D. Shah, S.T. Amann, J.J. Karlitz, The time is now: a guide to sustainable telemedicine during COVID-19 and beyond. Am. J. Gastroenterol. **115**(9), 1371–1375 (2020)
68. T.C.T. Chen, M.C. Chiu, Evaluating the sustainability of smart technology applications in healthcare after the COVID-19 pandemic: a hybridising subjective and objective fuzzy group decision-making approach with explainable artificial intelligence. Digital Health **8**, 20552076221136380 (2022)
69. G.G. Sagaro, G. Battineni, F. Amenta, Barriers to sustainable telemedicine implementation in Ethiopia: a systematic review. Telemed. Rep. **1**(1), 8–15 (2020)
70. T.C.T. Chen, in *Sustainable Smart Healthcare: Lessons Learned from the COVID-19 Pandemic.* Evaluating the Sustainability of a Smart Healthcare Application (2023), pp. 39–63
71. C. Combi, B. Amico, R. Bellazzi, A. Holzinger, J.H. Moore, M. Zitnik, J.H. Holmes, A manifesto on explainability for artificial intelligence in medicine. Artif. Intell. Med. **133**, 102423 (2022)
72. T. Chen, Y.C. Wang, A two-stage explainable artificial intelligence approach for classification-based job cycle time prediction. Int. J. Adv. Manuf. Technol. **123**(5–6), 2031–2042 (2022)

73. Y.C. Lin, T.C.T. Chen, An intelligent system for assisting personalized COVID-19 vaccination location selection: Taiwan as an example. Digital Health **8**, 20552076221109064 (2022)
74. M. Wan, N. Shukla, J. Li, B. Pradhan, Optimization of teleconsultation appointment scheduling in National Telemedicine Center of China. Comput. Ind. Eng. **183**, 109492 (2023)
75. T.C.T. Chen, in *Explainable Artificial Intelligence (XAI) in Manufacturing: Methodology, Tools, and Applications.* Applications of XAI to Job Sequencing and Scheduling in Manufacturing (2023), pp. 83–105
76. S.A. Erdogan, T.L. Krupski, J.M. Lobo, Optimization of telemedicine appointments in rural areas. Serv. Sci. **10**(3), 261–276 (2018)
77. T. Chen, M.C. Chiu, A fuzzy collaborative intelligence approach to group decision-making: a case study of post-COVID-19 restaurant transformation. Cogn. Comput. **14**(2), 531–546 (2022)
78. Y.C. Wang, T. Chen, Adapted techniques of explainable artificial intelligence for explaining genetic algorithms on the example of job scheduling. Expert Syst. Appl. **237**(A), 121369 (2024)
79. A.B. Cengil, B. Eksioglu, S. Eksioglu, H. Eswaran, C.J. Hayes, C.A. Bogulski, Using data analytics for telehealth utilization: a case study in Arkansas. J. Telemed. Telecare 1357633X231160039 (2023)
80. T. Chen, Y.C. Wang, Recommending suitable smart technology applications to support mobile healthcare after the COVID-19 pandemic using a fuzzy approach. Healthcare **9**(11), 1461 (2021)
81. A.E. Loeb, S.S. Rao, J.R. Ficke, C.D. Morris, L.H. Riley III., A.S. Levin, Departmental experience and lessons learned with accelerated introduction of telemedicine during the COVID-19 crisis. J. Am. Acad. Orthop. Surg. **28**(11), e469–e476 (2020)